PILLOW TALK

AN AWFULLY HILARIOUS ANTHOLOGY

Pillow Talk

REAL PEOPLE
REAL STORIES
REAL AWKWARD

Edited by
Angelina Jimenez & Heather Hendrie

Published by Awfully Hilarious Books
An imprint of Tidewater Press
New Westminster, BC, Canada
tidewaterpress.ca

978-1-990160-67-7 (print)
978-1-990160-68-4 (e-book)

An earlier version of "Panty Vending Machine" by Sophia McGovern was performed at the Erotic Poetry and Music Festivus at Alwun House, Phoenix, Arizona in 2018.

LIBRARY AND ARCHIVES CANADA CATALOGUING IN PUBLICATION
Title: Pillow talk : real people, real stories, real awkward / edited by Angelina Jimenez and Heather Hendrie.
Other titles: Pillow talk (2026)
Names: Jimenez, Angelina, editor. | Hendrie, Heather, editor.
Description: "An Awfully Hilarious anthology."
Identifiers: Canadiana (print) 2025031505X | Canadiana (ebook) 20250315114 | ISBN 9781990160677 (softcover) | ISBN 9781990160684 (EPUB)
Subjects: LCSH: Sex—Anecdotes. | LCSH: Sex—Humor.
Classification: LCC HQ21 .P55 2026 | DDC 306.7—dc23

Canadä

Tidewater Press gratefully acknowledges the support of the Government of Canada.

Contents

. . . the bridge which connects [the spiritual and the political] is formed by the erotic—the sensual—those physical, emotional, and psychic expressions of what is deepest and strongest and richest within each of us, being shared: the passions of love, in its deepest meanings.

AUDRE LORDE
Uses of the Erotic: The Erotic as Power, 1978

Foreword

ANGELINA JIMENEZ & HEATHER HENDRIE

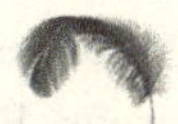

CONTENT NOTE

Grown-up themes ahead—intimacy, desire, and the vulnerable bits. Not for younger readers. Read gently, at your own pace.

Thank you so much for being here! You've (perhaps unwittingly) now joined our fast-growing community of folks ready to get real, and thus help normalize the messy, awkward, awfully hilarious experience of being human.

Have you ever sat with a friend over coffee to unpack your latest sex-capade gone wrong (or maybe oooooh-so right) then walked away feeling lighter and happier, having laughed harder than you thought was possible? Well, we have, and we realize just how freeing and healing those stigma-smashing conversations can be. We believe that one of the greatest (and most joyous) ways to undermine harmful narratives is through storytelling and humor. So, in a society that tells us not to talk about sex, intimacy, or pleasure (despite TLC telling us they wanted to "talk about sex, baby!"), we decided to tackle the taboo.

Writing real stories about sex isn't only about putting pleasure on the page; it's about giving readers and writers an opportunity to connect with the sensual sides of themselves and each other. Exploring erotic pleasure goes beyond sex to something much deeper—the vitality of being human and allowing our senses to open up to the world around us. To let in joy and pleasure, beyond what happens between the sheets. The erotic has long been stigmatized, feared, and locked behind closed doors, not because it is wrong, but because it is such a potent force. As we deepen our capacity to feel in all aspects of life, we begin to experience true empowerment. From this place, we regain access to belonging and connection, those aspects of life so necessary to our thriving.

Sex isn't a bad word; eroticism isn't sinful. But we've been conditioned to believe that they are. Overcoming that conditioning takes strength and courage. The authors in this anthology have demonstrated both, making themselves vulnerable and sharing their experiences with sex, intimacy, pleasure, and love (or lack thereof). It's their way of offering a shared space for joy, healing, community, and perhaps most importantly, laughter.

It became clear from the moment we issued our call for submissions that our community was exploding with desire: desire to belong, share, connect, love, and be loved. Generosity and the desire to share show up in each of these stories. As our writers open their hearts to you, we hope that in receiving their words, you will realize that connection, community, and support are much more available than you may have thought. This book is an act of care for our community, not because we're talking about a stigmatized topic, but because it has allowed us to stand in our strength and courage with hands outstretched to folks around the world.

In fact, this book was birthed by community. It was thanks to the generous donors of our Kickstarter campaign that this book came to be (you know who you are) and—can you believe it—our *69th* backer brought us over the finish line! Ha, but of course! Thank you all for making this book possible.

To be able to share our stories with one another and with our readers as we work together to heal our relationships with sex, intimacy, and pleasure has been our great privilege. We are honored to share these pages with authors from a variety of backgrounds. Where possible, and when there were choices to be made, we have prioritized stories by people from cultures or countries that have been censored or marginalized in mainstream publishing.

Pillow Talk seeks to unlock the doors of pleasure, intimacy, and joy; to begin mending our relationships with the erotic, to find love for ourselves and others where we never thought possible. Thank you, dear reader, for being here with us. Your participation in this community gives us the permission to share our stories, and to find pleasure and humor where we'd least expect it. Saying yes (or moaning it!) creates an opportunity to start conversations and build community once the book has closed and the cup of coffee or tea has cooled.

With all our sexy, sassy, sensual, saucy, earth-shaking, and sometimes steamy love,

Angelina & Heather

Ménage à Moi

JADE FRANCESCA BARTLETT

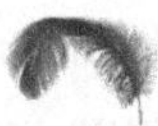

Having a wank shouldn't be *this* hard. But—alas! I am a twenty-five-year-old virgin[1] and still living with my parents. What is a tactile act of self-love for those who have the privilege of living alone is, for me, a *tactical* act of "don't let anyone catch ya."

To masturbate, I must remind myself of the following steps:

1. Bring up a clean towel from the laundry room into your bedroom.
2. Unearth your vibrator[2] from its hiding place (top

1. The writer would like to note that when she first wrote this piece, she was, in fact, a twenty-five-year-old virgin. However, due to a miraculous—and homoerotic—turn of events, she has since lost her virginity to her current partner, whom she loves to the moon and back then twice around!
2. The mighty rabbit, dressed to the nines in Royal Purple—because this pussy is QUEEN!

shelf of the closet, sandwiched between two piles of books, and concealed in an empty Quality Street tin from two Decembers ago).

3. Wrap the vibrator in the towel before exiting your bedroom and making your way across the hall to the bathroom.
4. Before doing *anything else,* lock the door.
5. Double-check the door is *actually* locked.
6. *Triple*-check the door is *actually* locked (you mustn't forget the time your younger sister, who has no regard for the privacy of others, almost caught you in the act—spread eagle, too!).
7. Once the door is *definitely* locked, wash the vibrator with warm water and unscented soap (scented soap will make your coochie itch[3]) and then rinse it thoroughly. You wouldn't want to start queefing soap bubbles now, would you?
8. Turn on the bathroom fan—its whirring will be necessary to mask the sound of you revving up your vibrator to the highest setting. Think . . . a jackhammer on Adderall.
9. Turn off the lights. This way, if your sister decides

3. However, venereal itching caused by scented soap could never hold a light to the venereal burning caused by lube that "heats up." Before using lube of this variety, it is important to read the warning label *before* diving in. I repeat: EXTERNAL USE ONLY.

to pick the lock because she needs her hairbrush, the darkness will provide a few crucial seconds to assume a more . . . *wholesome* pose in the bathtub.

10. Get into the tub and make sure you turn on the faucet before you turn on the vibrator—the more background noise, the better!
11. Now, this is where things get a little ~~sticky~~. Oh! Um, I meant *tricky*.
12. See, you mustn't push down the drain stopper quite yet because: a) the water will wash away all the lube, be it vaginal fluid, from a bottle, or a little bit of both. And honey, I'm telling you, there's nothing pleasurable about a dry wank; b) one might not necessarily "finish" by the time the bathtub has filled up. Ergo, you would have to turn off the water. No running water means no sound to mask you buzzing away, which means you'll have to prematurely pull the rabbit from the . . . hat. And, really, what's a magician without her magic wand?
13. So . . . y'gotta time it right. With the drain unplugged, let the faucet run for five minutes, seven max. Then, push the drain stopper down. Should all go well, you'll be able to *ménage à moi* yourself to ecstasy with no interruptions! By the time the water reaches your lower shins, you'll be right on the verge of an—Oh! Oh! Oh!

14. Ohhhhhhhhhhhhhhhhhhhhhhhhhhhhhhhhhhhhhhhh hhhhhhhhhhhhhhrgasm.
15. Ah, that's better!

Rhymes With Tennis

GEOFFREY K. GRAVES

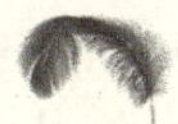

In the 1960s, an eighth-grade biology class was far more rudimentary than what is taught today. Mr. Peters (not his real name) was our biology teacher at Wilhelmina C. Peabody Junior High School (not its real name) in Santa Sabinas (ditto), California (real). In the lab section of the class, students outfitted with goggles, protective bibs, and scalpels were tasked with dissecting earthworms and frogs. Yuck.

I had no idea what future value there might be in performing such procedures, and if there ever happened to be such a job opening, I doubt it would have paid much. Except for a few weirdos, most of us didn't want to dissect anything. Where was PETA when you needed them? I have yet to perform another autopsy, but heard on National Public Radio that these procedures survive in schools today. Pity the lowly earthworm, mourn the doomed frog.

Truth be told, worm or frog anatomy was of minor importance to us kids because older brothers, sisters, and friends had already tipped us off about a far more intriguing lecture to come—one that was the highlight of eighth-grade biology. From Day One, each of us waited for revelation moment when two diagram charts above the chalkboard would be unfurled. They taunted us the entire semester, curled up in spring-loaded tension behind Mr. Peters. Would he ever get on with it? He was, evidently, saving the best for last.

Peters was a soft-spoken man who always wore a crisp white lab coat. Grade A testosterone must have run in his family because he had one of the thickest five o'clock shadows I've ever seen, his dark stubble blue-black. Whenever he lectured, Peters waved a wooden pointer with a black rubber tip on the end, clutched tightly like an adult security blanket.

As days became weeks, then months, we all wondered what in the world he was waiting for. Finally, one week before the final exam, time was up. Revelation day had arrived. The class was giddy, wound up as tight as the charts, each of us barely able to contain ourselves. As junior high schoolers, hormonally speaking, we were at our pubescent fever pitch.

It soon became apparent why Peters had been stalling: he was as nervous about the lesson as we were. He took forever, over-embroidering explanations he'd already given until slowly, finally, he unrolled chart Number One: an illustration of the female anatomy. On the left side of her body, the woman was shown with skin on, naked. On the right, her innards were displayed.

Peters' mouth went dry. He sipped a glass of water, then with trusty pointer in hand, started at the top of the female figure telling us things we already knew: nasal passages, tear ducts, larynx, and so on. He finally got down to the breasts and, speaking in a slow, emotionless monotone, said, "These are the breasts." Another sip. "There are two of them. One on the left. One on the right. Side-by-side. As you can see." Sip-sip. "There are glands in the breasts capable of producing milk to feed an infant. And here," he tapped the pointer on the chart, "we discover the areola which surrounds the nipple that expresses the milk I just mentioned."

"Mr. Peters, I have a question about the nipples," piped up one brave youth. "Does one of the nipples express chocolate milk and the other vanilla? My brother told me that was true."

Peters took a breath, narrowed his eyes a bit trying to figure out if Robin was being serious or having him on, then remembered something. He said, "No, Mr. Graham, that is not true, as your brother knows perfectly well because he asked that same question three years ago in this very class, as I suspect you know. Now, then . . ."

Emboldened by Robin's question, John Kulish weighed in. "Mr. Peters, two questions. First, is the milk from the nipple the same as cow milk?"

"No, Mr. Kulish, it is chemically different. What's your other question?"

"What's the purpose of the areola?"

"The purpose of the areola is . . . well, I really don't know. Perhaps you can research that and do an extra-credit report for us. Now, class, please hold your questions until I have finished. Where was I, the arm tits? Pits! I meant pits, darn it!"

Tittering from the class took a while to die down. "You were starting on the areolas," Debbie Utley, one of the sharper students, said, guiding Peters back on track.

"Thank you, Deborah, you've put your finger on it. I mean, yes, we were on the areolas." Tap-tap-tap went Peters' pointer, as though he'd developed a palsy. He took a deep breath and continued. "There are two areolas. One per breast. There are two nipples. One per areola." Peters worked his tongue in his mouth in search of any saliva. Failing that, he started up again with the sipping and swallowing routine, but it was no good. As he got more nervous, we got more nervous, the tension in the air thickening.

The pointer tapped its way down the diagram until, with quivering voice, Peters squeaked, "This is the pubis area." He swallowed hard, as though a lump of the cafeteria's dry roast beef was stuck in his throat. He loosened his black tie. Same black tie every day. "And this is the va-, va-, va-," tappity-tap-tap, " . . .gina."

I thought Peters was going to pass out. He hadn't even unrolled the male chart yet, and sweat was dripping down his blue-black sideburns. He could barely keep his pointer on the chart.

He finished with the woman, rolled up that chart with a sharp snap, and slowly drew down the male chart, again beginning at the top. Hair, scalp, eyebrows, eyeballs, brain, cerebral cortex, etcetera. After dawdling several more minutes, he arrived at the male privates, the wobbling pointer producing sharp whap-whap-whaps against the chart.

Finally, it was too much for him. He turned, grabbed his water glass, took too big a gulp, and coughed, spraying it all over the chart. He pretended to accidentally drop his pointer, took a long moment to bend over, breathe, and regroup. As he came up, he surreptitiously tried to swipe the chart with the arm of his lab coat, completely missing. As he continued, the water rolled down in rivulets, puddling on the floor.

Peters fanned his face with his pointer-free hand. "Whew. Warm day." He smiled weakly and moved over to the thermostat, where he turned on the AC full blast.

This may sound like some cock-and-bull story, but none of it is invention. Any kid who was in that class talked about it for years. I'm still talking about it, and I'm old. This guy was freaking out. He steadied his pointer with both hands, placed the rubber tip on the man's pouch, and with a robot-like voice, said, "This is the scro-tum. And inside the scro-tum," he pointed at the gonads, "are the testicles," which he pronounced tess-tee-culz. His perspiration had now created two large rings under the armpits of his lab coat. "There are two tess-tee-culz. One on the right side. One on the left. These tess-tee-culz are what produce see-men, a liquid filled with spermatozoa which, uh, once planted, seek out the egg in the female that eventually grows into a baby."

"Question about the planting," Robin Graham tried, his expression angelic, his intent devilish.

"Can it, Graham!" Peters exploded, whipping out a handkerchief from his lab coat pocket to blot his glistening forehead and the beads of moisture that had formed on his stubbled upper lip.

Every kid in the room was about to lose it. I caught a glimpse of the girl to my right, whose face was red. She peeked at me at the same time; we both gave each other a look that said, "Can you believe this guy?" In a feeble attempt at self-control, we clamped our hands over our mouths.

The whole room was throbbing with suppressed energy like Poe's telltale heart as the pointer moved ever closer to the you-know-what. Finally, Peters got up the gumption and placed the black tip on the illustrated man's member. The pointer went crazy. It was as if our teacher had been hit with a 220-volt live wire, causing the pointer to produce an impressive series of loud whap-whap-whaps like a flag in a hurricane. The moment had at last arrived. The entire room held its collective breath.

Then, Mr. Peters said something I will never forget. "And this . . ." (lick dry lips) ". . . is the man's pennis."

That is not a typo. Pennis. Not penis. Pennis. And our biology teacher did not know how to say it. Every kid in the class was ready to hear penis, but Peters said pennis. Rhymes with tennis. Pennis.

By the eighth grade, you've pretty much got down the names of the private parts of the human anatomy. Children say they have to pee-pee, not pen-pen. Peters' pronunciation had us all perplexed, though there was one thing good about the *pennis* pronunciation. It deflated the nervousness out of us kids. Imagine one big thought bubble floating over the classroom that said, "Huh?!" We were all stumped because if anybody should know how to say the word, the biology teacher would be that guy, right? I was wondering if I'd had it wrong all along.

Well, Peters timed it perfectly because the bell rang right after the pennis had been described. He yanked that chart so hard it fell onto the floor, where some internal spring tried to roll itself back up. Class was dismissed.

There were some interesting conversations in the hallway afterward, and some interesting conversations around dinner tables that night. Here's how it went at my house:

ME: Hey, Pops, you know what you told me my thingy is called?

POPS: (Shooting a look at my mother) . . . Yeeesssssss.

ME: Are you sure it's called that?

POPS: Why do you ask?

ME: Well, Mr. Peters gave us the biology lecture today about male and female anatomy, and when he got to the middle of the man chart, he put his pointer on the dick and called it a pennis.

POPS: A what? And don't use the dick term in front of your mother and sister.

ME: He called it a pennis.

POPS: Pennis?

ME: Yep, pennis.

POPS: He's nuts.

ME: No, he called them tess-tee-culz.

POPS: No, I mean he is looney tunes. It is called penis. Not pennis.

ME: You sure?

POPS: I am sure.

ME: But he is a biology teacher. How do you know your parents didn't tell you wrong and you passed on bad info to me?

POPS: Lookit. Peters doesn't know his nuts from his hat. I know it is a penis. Your mom knows it is a penis. Her parents told her it is a penis. Right?

MOM: Yes.

POPS: It is a penis. Penis-penis-penis. Hear me? If you want to call it a pennis, go ahead, but everybody's going to laugh you out of the building.

ME: Okay. Is a vagina called a vagina?

POPS: Yep. Now, take your little pennis and go do the dishes.

ME: Okay. That was pretty funny, Pops.

POPS: Right. Dishes.

As I cleared the table, my father said to my mother, "That school needs a new biology teacher. Pennis!"

Young, Hot, & Infertile

CLAIRE LOCEY

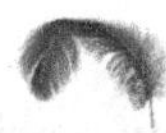

"I'm ovulating," I whisper to my husband.

This used to be a primal turn-on. Now, it's the bane of my existence.

My husband and I have been trying to conceive for the past year, which, if you like statistics or excessive Googling (like me), makes me a fertility failure compared to 85% of women who try to conceive. Not to mention, I am the ripe age of twenty-six. I know . . . young, hot, and allegedly fertile, right?

Ironically, I am a women's health nerd, so I have been doing all the "right" things from the get-go: tracking my basal body temperature every morning, taking the ovulation tests, and, best of all, eliminating every last ounce of sparkle from my life.

Don't drink caffeine on an empty stomach; it'll ruin

your hormones. Don't go into a sauna or a hot tub or a cold tub. Don't exercise too hard. But also exercise every day . . . for your hormones. And don't drink alcohol. Or eat sugar. Or eat too much. Or too little. All together now: For! Your! Hormones!

Fun fact about me and my reproductive system: I have something called *Mittelschmerz,* which is a stupid fucking German name for "extremely painful ovulation." This is my best evidence that God, sadly, is not a woman. Sorry. There's just no way she'd greenlight such a thing.

Mittelschmerz means, every month, I present myself to my husband like a beached, bloated whale with stabbing pain in whatever useless ovary is releasing the egg that month.

I try to make it sexy. But nothing about me feels sexy these days, and I spend a lot of time crying in my car.

Very teen angst of me, I know. But, having been on synthetic hormones for years, I haven't had a natural cycle since I was thirteen, okay? And it's like I am going through puberty all over again, only now I have adult responsibilities. And I can't take it out on my mom because I have matured and come to realize that my mom's an angel.

In case you're wondering, my favorite crying-in-the-car song is "So Hard," from my favourite band, The

Chicks, which laments about being a woman struggling with fertility.

Back when I was in school, I never really knew what I wanted to be when I grew up. I was good at sciences; I loved writing. I took the LSAT because I come from a family of lawyers but studied for and received a Master of Science and a Bachelor of Arts in Gender and Women's Studies instead.

But one thing I have known in my heart and soul since forever is that I wanted to be a mom one day. I have been mesmerized by pregnancy, sexuality, and womanhood my whole life. Which is why I wrote my master's thesis on women's healthcare experiences at the intersection of pregnancy and homelessness, which now feels like a sick joke.

And on top of that, I *love* love. I love romance and admire the commitment of being with someone forever and building a life together. To me, making a baby is a rare moment in life where all these things collide. Feminism hasn't always made space for women who dream of motherhood, but this dream has always been mine, and it doesn't make me any less of a strident feminist, I promise. This experience, however, has been the opposite of how I always imagined it and has left me feeling like I've lost my faith. Hey Siri, add, "Losing My Religion" by R.E.M. to my crying-in-the-car playlist.

This loss of faith seems odd considering I am not a religious person, and I don't really know what my faith was before. I think I believed in the timing of the Universe and Mother Nature and love and karma and energy. Maybe I was just a fairy or a witch. But lately, it feels like all those beliefs have been sucked out of me. The vulnerability and desperation that come with the experience of infertility have brought me to my knees. Praying, yearning, and, of course, scream-crying in my car for things to be different.

With that said, my favorite part of this unexpected and difficult time in my life has been having an excessive amount of erotic, beautiful, passionate sex. And I mean a *lot* of it. Even with the ovulation-day pain. My husband and I quickly realized, though, that despite how romantic the notion may be, the quality of the sex does not correlate with conception. Unfortunately. Because if making a baby was determined by how good the sex was or how much we loved each other, I would be pregnant all the time.

Despite our tantric "trying," every passing month feels like a cycle of building hope, then getting my heart broken over and over again by my own body. Then having to put the pieces of myself back together to do it all over again the following month, all the while bleeding from my vagina.

After our first appointment at the fertility clinic, my husband turned to me and said, "So let me get this straight. You have to get poked and prodded and go through so much suffering, and all I have to do is come in a cup?"

The tension and irony of this pleasure-pain dichotomy is not lost on us. Like I said, there is no way that God is a woman.

I am exhausted from feeling like every month is Groundhog Day. And from forcing myself to feel hopeful just because a little strip I peed on told me it's my *perfect moment*.

So, tonight, I will light a candle, and I will, yet again, try to mask my bloated and joy-free existence with whatever sexy charade I can muster while whispering seductively that I am ovulating. Because this, apparently, is the erotically complicated pinnacle of my twenties. And I'll keep peeing on sticks, seducing my sweet husband on cue, and crying in my car to a playlist curated by heartbreak and hormones. Not because it's romantic, but because it's real.

Because maybe it's not magic or faith I need right now, but the rawness itself. And the honesty it holds.

Tuning Guitars and Wet Kisses

NICOLE BREIT & CLAIRE SICHERMAN

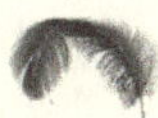

Dear Claire,

When I read your recent letter, I had an epiphany.

You know how Virginia Woolf says that in order to write, women need a room of their own? Well, for women to experience sexual pleasure, we need solitude to explore our sensations and to believe we deserve it. In other words, we need to find a way to override centuries of internalized shame.

That's right. Whatever you've got stashed in your bedside drawer shouldn't be the stuff of whispers or shamed silence. I want to live in a world where female fantasies are shared and celebrated, knowing winks over moist morning panties as commonplace as teenage boy jokes about jizz T-shirts and tube socks.

I still recall my first sexy dream. It was about my

brother's catechism teacher: a tall, suited man with messy blond hair. When he slid into his pew with his wife and young child, I couldn't stop looking at him. My eyes kept landing on his square jaw. When he passed the collection plate, I'd drop some coins in and register the blueness of his eyes—then a wave would radiate through my body, my skin itchy with heat.

This man was in his late twenties, and I was a girl, yet I'd dreamed I'd been with him in the grass along the side of my house. I was me and not me. Somehow, there I was, ten years older, wearing a black lacy thing like the negligees I'd seen in the Sears catalogue, with a soft, curvy woman's body to match.

During junior high, I was often struck out of nowhere by a sudden awareness of my pulse in my most private place. So that I couldn't be accused of touching myself (or later have to confront our red-faced, bulbous-nosed parish priest who reeked of whiskey in the confessional), I never did so directly. Instead, I'd lock the bathroom door and lie on the cool tile, close my eyes, and think of nothing and no one. When I held my breath and moved just the right way, there was rushing in my ears, then a hot flush across my cheeks, then strange waves deep in my core—a rhythmic opening and closing so intense it made my breath catch.

The rushing and the waves and the calm feeling after

helped my anxious mind relax, but everything I did to make that happen was my secret. I felt weird, and shameful, and confused that something that felt good could be wrong. I was sure I was the only girl at my school who committed this sin of the flesh. At night, I'd ask God to make me stop, but my body's desire for sensation overruled my will.

When God didn't give me the strength to stop having orgasms, I began to rationalize that I could not be the only girl bent this way. I scanned the innocent faces of my Grade 8 homeroom to guess who the other female perverts were. (No need to compare myself with the boys: they were all perverts.) I suspected the wholesome straight-A student athlete with pretty brown curls who never wore makeup. I think I decided she was actually normal—not a deviant like me—even if it turned out she did masturbate, because it was okay for non-Catholic girls to get sexy however they wanted.

Girls who didn't go to catechism didn't have to worry about going to Hell. They could re-read the good parts from *Flowers in the Attic* under the sheets by flashlight. Or sneak peeks at a *Playboy* tucked inside a Teen Beat at Soupy's corner store. Lie naked in bed while unzipping Wonder Woman's costume or sliding a hand up Princess Leia's leg along the slit in her long white skirt. Make out with two cute boys who looked like Corey Haim and Matt Dillon in the gully behind their house.

I'd heard the words "vibrator" and "dildo," uttered with a pervy grin by the slobby D-student with a fuzzy moustache who flashed his porn stash at me from under his coat during silent reading in sixth grade. But sex toys, I knew, were for depraved women—the stuff of jokes.

In college, a decade later, I complained to a friend about the extent of my horniness, to which she replied, "Well, you do have two hands." A lapsed Catholic, had she been locking herself in her bathroom and holding her breath, too? Or was there really nothing wrong with pleasure, and I was the last to know?

In the late 90s, a poster of Kurt Cobain replaced the painting of Jesus above my bed in my studio apartment. Under Kurt's watch, I wrote my first song on acoustic guitar for a shaggy artist who couldn't love me back. I wrote another one for my future wife. I'd come out by then and was beginning to deconstruct my childhood religious shame. Still, I was surprised when I joked to a friend about what I called "tuning my guitar." She chuckled and asked, "Doesn't everyone do it?"

Uh, no one talked about it so . . . how would I know?

Fast forward twenty-five years. This past summer, I took on a sexy pleasure project: with agreement from my wife, I connected with men on dating apps to chat about desires and fantasies. Dipping my toes into ethical non-monogamy as a married bisexual woman, I was back to a question that kept me up at night as a teen: how would a consensual sexual encounter even start?

My best conversations were with two guys in their mid-to-late thirties—roughly fifteen years younger than me. One was pansexual, one straight, each attractive to me in their own ways. I was delighted by the vulnerability they brought to our conversations and surprised by how focused they were on my pleasure as an end in itself—without expectation, without asking for more. One of my favorite exchanges was with Daniel, who told me he liked my eyes and that he would really like to seduce me. I was game for him to try, but a bit skeptical. Wasn't seduction about tuning in? How could he sense what I wanted over an app?

Together we imagined the people in our profile photos—the tall man with the trimmed beard in the suit and skinny tie, and the woman in the silver-sequined party dress and heels—meeting in person. He painted a scene for me alive with sensory detail, charged with erotic energy, each subtle shift so attuned to what I'd want that it felt like he was drawing imagery straight from my own mind. The distance didn't matter. We had chemistry.

"Are you a writer?" I messaged. "You're very good at this!"

"Thank you," he replied. "It helps to have such beautiful inspiration."

Seduction isn't just about tuning in. It's about pacing, too. I loved that this man was in no rush as he described his next move and each embodied response. He was seducing me, alright. Belly tingling, ears ringing, I couldn't stop myself from urging him on to the chorus.

"Can I tell you what I want?" I dared to ask.

"Please tell me what you want."

So I did. And he gave it to me in a paragraph I've since read over and over again. And yes, yes, it was good.

Say what you will about dating apps, isn't it something that a stranger who lives a thousand miles away opened me up to aspects of my sexuality I'd allowed to wither over the years?

A large part of recovering my authentic self has meant embracing that women deserve to experience pleasure in any way that feels good. I believe the only sin committed in my young Catholic life was the imposition of rules that suppressed my vast capacity for self-expression and love. And that it took me until the age of fifty to return to the acknowledgment and fulfillment of my desires.

So, Claire, I can't wait for your next letter and the stories about your high school years you haven't yet told me—about desire, pleasure, or any subject you'd like to share.

Your kindred spirit in late awakenings,

Nicole

xo

Dear Nicole,

I was elated after reading your last letter, a huge smile on my face as I learned about your pleasure project. At the same time, I wanted to reach out and hug your younger self. How confusing it must have been for you—the intensity of an orgasm, followed by the feeling you've done something terribly wrong.

I don't remember when I first felt that intensity in my own body, but I didn't understand it, which meant that it was scary. It was around this time, when my body was rapidly changing and attracting unwanted comments from boys and men, that I began to hide. I wore baggy clothing and retreated into myself: a once confident and boisterous girl, gone quiet. All I knew was that this feeling, this heat, this wave, this vibration, was something else I needed to tamp down. But I wonder what would have happened if I had allowed myself to experience it fully? Girls and women are labeled sluts if we act on our desires and frigid if we don't. We are pressured to say yes even if we want to say no.

Up until then, my experience with bodies came from books. My parents left me with copies of *Where Did I Come From?* and the follow-up, *What's Happening to Me?*, by Peter Mayle. I was hooked, swept up in cartoons of people in their birthday suits, my nether regions stirring slightly as I flipped through the pages.

My only experience of real, live naked humans was when my parents accidentally took us to Wreck Beach in Vancouver when I was twelve. My parents didn't realize we were on a nude beach until my friend Sandra pointed and yelled, "I can see her boobs!"

Witnessing not one but two naked men in one day for the first time in my life is something I still can't erase from my mind. There was the tall, pale, thin, elderly man with a fancy top hat, black socks pulled up his shins, dress shoes, and nothing else. The other man was moustached and hairy à la Burt Reynolds. He sat on a towel, shades on and legs spread. I tried to avert my eyes, but I also wanted to look, and experienced the same conflict you described in your letter.

My first cassette tape was the soundtrack to the movie *Dirty Dancing*. When I was older, I watched Patrick Swayze in a black tank top and tight black pants, biceps bulging. When he and Jennifer Grey moved across the dance floor, crotches connected, I began to feel a gentle pulse in my own.

Around this time, I hung out with the neighborhood boys who lived across the street. In the summers, we'd smear dish soap on our bellies and fly across their orange, water-soaked Sundance trampoline; in the winters, we'd launch snowballs at cars from our fort. I was the oldest and one day decided it was time to play "I'll show you mine if you show me yours." I knew what I had going on down there, and I was curious what they had.

One by one, the boys showed me theirs. But instead of showing mine, I darted across the street and back into the safety of my home. My pubic hair had begun to sprout, and since theirs hadn't yet, I felt too ashamed to show them.

My poor excuse for sex education continued with junior high science class. Mr. M was given the task of teaching us about the birds and the bees, and he did this in two ways. The first was by telling us stories about his sexual escapades with his wife. I don't remember what he said. I'm sure I've blocked it from my memory because . . . Eww! Gross!

The second way he "taught" us was through videos of animals having sex. From lionesses and leopardesses to cows and hens, there wasn't one female animal who looked like she was deriving any pleasure from sex. Typically, the male would overpower the female, mount and have his way with her, while the female desperately tried to escape. After he finished (which was usually pretty quickly), the male would roll over and fall asleep. Was this foreshadowing what I could look forward to?

In eighth grade, I decided I had a crush on Nick, a red-headed, freckled boy who walked like he had a pole stuck up his ass. I heard that he liked me, so I pretended to like him back. Having a boy who liked me gave me a certain status. I felt more popular (even though I wasn't) and beautiful (ditto). And then, at a school dance, after we finished grooving to C+C Music Factory's "Gonna Make You Sweat," and swaying to the last song of the night, Boyz II Men's "End of the Road," we kissed.

The kiss happened so fast, like a blink—it was literally the smallest, wettest peck on the lips. A second later, Nick disappeared back into the boy huddle on one side of the gym, and I darted into the hallway, where I waited for my mom to pick me up.

My first real kiss happened with Theo when we were both seventeen. I felt an electricity with Theo that I hadn't with Nick. Yet that kiss felt strange to me, all lips and spit with our tongues and teeth getting in the way. Slippery, too. Hard to breathe. After all, mouths were food portals, not pleasure centers! And what were we supposed to do with our noses? But I got used to it. And pretty soon, I enjoyed it.

When I met my husband, Jeremy, we went out on one of those epic first all-day dates. One where you start in the late afternoon and wind up walking all over the city talking, and forgetting about inconsequential things like time and eating and peeing. It's just the two of you together, and nothing else exists. When we kissed for the first time, it was in the front seat of his black GMC. With my lips pressed against his, I didn't think about anything except my heart, which was hammering so hard I thought he could surely hear it.

A few months later, we were sitting on Jeremy's beige checkered couch, talking about our first date.

"Your kiss was so forceful and urgent it felt like you were going to eat my face off," he said.

I burst out laughing, cheeks flush with embarrassment.

It still makes me smile when I think about how, almost twenty-five years ago, I was kissing with such passion that he didn't know what to do with me.

Nicole, after that first kiss with Jeremy, I finally understood something about myself. There was nothing wrong with me all those years ago when I felt no desire for Nick. Tuning into the absence of desire may be just as important as desire itself.

With all my wet kissy love,

xo Claire

Into the Wild

HANNAH DAVIS

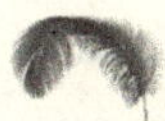

Madison lifted her arm overhead and swept her glossy black hair in front of her shoulder, where it fell in long, wild bunches down to her chest.

As she leaned against the arm of the sofa, the afternoon sun streamed through rustic white windows, lighting her up like some kind of film star. She laughed at something on TV—we were watching *Notting Hill*—and flashed me a big smile, setting a stream of colorful fireworks popping in my chest. It was all I could do not to stare at her constantly, with Care Bear love beams shooting out of my eyes.

I knew Madison had never been with a woman. Neither had I. I was in my early twenties and had dated a plethora of men without finding passion. I wondered if movies like this one had given me sky-high expectations and an unrealistic grip on reality. I knew how to tease, please, and perform—but wasn't there supposed to be more?

Madison reached out and began running her hand along my forearm. Innocently, the way she often did. I chewed my lip with a vengeance as the hairs on my neck prickled. She didn't know it—I had barely admitted it to myself—but I was in love with her.

Since we'd first met, a year earlier, I had imagined what her lips tasted like, over and over.One time, I'd admitted wanting to kiss her. She'd laughed it off, and I had wanted the ground to swallow me whole.

Gay people are wrong in the eyes of God and are doing something unnatural. My childhood pastor's words plagued my thoughts as I caught the scent of her perfume. Sitting on the couch with Madison didn't *feel* wrong.

Just as Hugh Grant was running a hand through his hair the way he does, before Julia Roberts kissed him at the front door, Madison shifted a little closer to me on the sofa and brushed her leg against mine. A rush moved up my chest.

We were petsitting and had not been in a situation like this before. Alone in a house together, uninterrupted. My eyes were trained on the screen, but I was no longer watching the movie. I could feel my heart beating in my ears.

Sitting in church with my parents, I had listened to the story of Adam and Eve, and how ashamed they were after realizing they were naked together in the Garden of Eden. My teenage self had squirmed thinking about Eve's body covered with only leaves. I shot a smirk at my best friend, wondering if she was intrigued, too. I doubted she was, because those were not thoughts we should be having.

"Would you like to sit between my legs so I can tickle both sides of your arms?" Madison asked.

I steeled myself as heat from her body surrounded me. Her hands moved on me like liquid ecstasy. I didn't know how much more of this I could take, my body now on fire. As I ran the backs of my fingers over her bare thigh, Madison took a sharp breath, and I felt her body shudder.

The sound of the TV hung suspended in the air as I stared blindly at the screen. *Am I imagining this?* With sudden courage, I leaned into Madison's chest. Seconds passed, but she didn't withdraw. Instead, she shifted my hair to the side with a delicate stroke and pressed her lips against my neck. My body became electrified. *I can't believe this is happening.*

Madison slid her hands under my white T-shirt and pressed them against my naked breasts, my skin like hot wax melting down a burning candle. *Surely Eve . . .*

would've approved of this . . . Madison moved so naturally, I wondered if I was dreaming.

I turned to face her. Her cheeks were flushed as she looked into my eyes, then at my mouth. Then she kissed me.

Women were not made to be with other women. That is the reason their body parts don't fit together. The dark voice I had listened to my whole life admonished me, but I couldn't deny myself this moment. I kissed her back, fully.

Heat poured off her as my fingers grazed her inner thigh, running along the seam of her shorts. Slipping my hand underneath, I ran my finger between her legs, and she let out a stifled moan. I used all my fingers to rub her and could feel the moist heat through her underwear. I wanted to make her come, to feel her body press against mine.

Madison took my hand and led me to the bedroom. A light breeze came through the open window as she stroked my arm with a little smile. Leaning forward, she touched her lips to mine, injecting me with something that felt like heaven. Her hair, her skin, her lips were everything I had been missing in my life.

Pushing me backwards, she threw a leg over my hips and pinned my arms over my head with a devilish grin. I could barely catch my breath as she moved down my body. She kissed, licked, and explored uninhibited, then knelt between my legs and hooked her fingers through my underwear, sliding them down my legs before flinging them across the room.

She swept her hair to the side again, and I glanced up at the ceiling. Nervously. Then I felt her tongue.

Pleasure reverberated up my body, my embarrassment swiftly vanishing. I clasped my hands together and pressed them into my forehead as I tried to process the intensity. Closing my eyes, I willed myself to believe that this was good, and right, and okay, even if deep down, my pastor's words pounded through my chest like a sledgehammer.

Madison licked me slowly and stroked my legs, all the way down to my feet, as I gripped the sheets. *How was everything about her so soft?* I felt her hair brushing my thighs and lifted my head as her fingers slid into me.

She paused and looked at me. "Would you like me to get your toys?"

"Really?" I laughed, unable to hide my grin. *She can't be serious.*

We knew all about each other's self-pleasure techniques. Madison slinked off to find them, reappearing minutes later with a handful of pink, silicone goodies. Falling onto the bed, she rolled back on top of me as I slid my hand down the curve of her back.

Masturbation is a blasphemous act. Homosexuality, an abomination—the words I had read as a teenager in a book gifted to my Sunday school class were still seared into my mind as if with a branding iron.

My eyes snapped open as I felt the toy penetrate me. She moved it in and out, and swirled her tongue over my clit, exploring new and different angles before sliding up my body to meet my mouth.

Madison handed me my little pink vibrator. In one movement, I felt her tongue in my mouth as she entered me with a slow thrust.

If this was the road to hell, I wanted to be on it.

She moved on me fluidly as her tongue alternated between licking my lips and plunging into my mouth. Slipping her hand under mine, she interlaced our fingers, filling me with a kind of love I didn't imagine possible.

Fighting tears, I squeezed my eyes shut and tipped fully into the most powerful orgasm I had ever known. I wasn't sure what spiritual enlightenment felt like, but I imagined it was something like this.

"Fucking hell!" I blurted out, as the sexual tension sizzled in the air. Eyes wide and chest heaving, my head spun with euphoria.

If you're having impure thoughts, take them to Jesus, and he will cleanse your mind. Thinking about the forbidden fruit was one thing, but *tasting* it was another. And now I had eaten that sexy fucking apple. *I am doomed.*

Madison and I hid in the shadows for what felt like a lifetime. Then, utterly consumed with anxiety—instead of accepting who I was, who I *am*—I ended our relationship and swore to take my secret to the grave.

Though I had other secret relationships with women throughout my late twenties, I often thought about that first time with Madison. How free and safe I had felt, how soft her skin was against mine, how her lips tasted when we kissed. The kind of kiss you wish would last forever. I remembered her breasts, her stomach, the freckle on her inner thigh. Looking between her legs, fascinated, as she smiled at me with her pink cheeks. The feeling of sliding my finger inside her and noticing how she felt just like me. Licking her slowly and watching in wonder as her back arched like a cat while I swept my hands over her most sensitive parts. She had looked like a goddess that night: her wild hair spilling over both pillows. When I came up to meet her mouth with my fingers still inside, she had pressed her forehead to mine and wrapped her legs around my waist. I had felt her nails clawing down my back, and hadn't stopped until she began to shake. I wanted to remember that moment forever—tasting her and feeling our bodies burning against the sheets— but could never escape the accompanying feeling of shame.

In my thirties, I began to worry I would never feel love like that again. Any relationships I had with women were at an arm's length; to allow my true feelings felt like a dangerous game.

Killing time on a flight to visit my family, I watched a movie called *Boy Erased*.

Based on a memoir by the closeted gay son of a pastor, the movie follows a young Christian man sent to a conversion camp. Seeing him endure the camp administrators' sickening attempts to straighten him out, I felt a knife twist in my gut. While he stood strong in the face of his parents' rejection and told them he wasn't going to change, I sobbed quietly in my seat, my seatbelt hugging my waist.

Seven years after Madison and I lay together—holding hands, staring at the ceiling, panting, dishevelled, delighted—I sat with my parents on their couch.

"Mom, Dad, I have something to tell you," I said, through a river of tears. The words wouldn't come out. *C'mon, you can do this. Please. God, help me do this.* I took a deep breath and prayed they would still love me. "I'm gay."

I shuddered with relief as the words floated from my mouth. *I was free.*

It took time, and many healing conversations, for my parents to embrace my sexuality. But I now feel truly accepted by them. More importantly, I have accepted myself. And that feels fucking glorious.

Jesus Take the Phone

SARAH BYRD

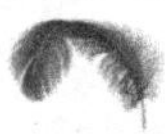

I'm not a particularly sexual person. I never really have been.

I'm not judgmental of others—as long as people are consenting adults, have fun! Do whatever you want. Be queer, be monogamous, or polyamorous. Be expressive, adventurous, wild, and crazy. Have all the sex you want! I'm happy for the great breadth and depth of human experience and expression, and have always believed diversity is a gift.

So have at it.

I just personally want to hang out on the sidelines instead of playing the field. I've never been one to enjoy crushes or be "boy crazy." To me, a crush is frustrating: I hate how the mental and emotional space for my own interests and projects gets pushed aside by some all-consuming focus on a person I may not even genuinely want. *Excuse me, here I was living in my own heart and mind, and some crush suddenly kicks me out because they've taken up residence instead.*

Even thinking about the elaborate dance of dating and finding someone I'm interested in makes me anxious. It's always such a lengthy process—trying to look "perfect" and hide all my flaws the first time we meet, nervously laughing too loudly at jokes that aren't even funny, trying to read every micro-expression to figure out if he's into me.

Not to mention all the stupid things people do to get attention. Like the time I bought a ticket to a beer festival so that I could casually run into a guy I liked. I don't even drink beer. And he didn't attend. But by God, I was ready to waste a Saturday hoping to run into a guy who barely knew I existed.

On those first few dates, I feel like I'm performing in some bad improv at a bar I didn't even want to go to in the first place, trying to guess what another person wants me to be. It all just feels so . . . inauthentic.

So, when a guy friend, someone I'd been loosely flirting with—smiling at his bad puns, lingering a beat too long when we said goodbye—called me up one night around 10:30 pm, I wasn't at all prepared for what was coming.

I met "Gary" (name changed, because God *forbid* he ever reads this) in a group therapy program for people going through breakups. My last relationship was a hot mess because I had no boundaries, and my ex-boyfriend loved people with no boundaries. Match made in hell.

Breakup group therapy is not an ideal place to meet men, I know. But that's where we met. As part of some group assignments, we'd had a few one-on-one video calls to talk through our breakups as therapy "homework." And we clicked.

Gary was not really my type—not my type at all, actually. A cowboy country-bumpkin who lives in rural Texas with his horses and chickens. The type of guy who wears his nice cowboy hat and best boots to make a trip into town for the rodeo. He had the brawn, but I'm a brains kinda gal.

So not in a million years would I have given him half a glance. Except for the fact he had the secret weapon to my romantic Achilles heel: He gave me the slightest, I mean *slightest*, amount of romantic attention.

I could see he tried to hide a smile that eventually slipped through whenever our therapy group talked on video. He looked at me when someone made a joke, and the whole screen of faces laughed. And he always seemed a little too eager to partner with me.

Now, I'm not desperate. I'm happily single and

have spent the majority of my adult life living alone. I genuinely enjoy my own company and having my own space. I'm an introvert, so I need lots of alone time anyway. I'm satisfied with solo life.

But when a man shows any interest in me, he activates my stupidity reflex—remember my beer festival adventure? It's like waking a sleeper agent who has no sense of self outside of the mission. When Gary called me up that night, it was my sleeper-agent self who interacted with him, not *me*.

I was taking a bubble bath and reading. First *and* second mistake, because I know better than to choose talking with a man rather than reading a good story. And I know better than to talk to a man while naked.

I shouldn't have even picked up, but when I did, I could already tell he was drunk. Third mistake: don't talk with people when they're drunk.

I knew that Gary had a crush on me and, like I said, I'd lightly flirted back and even entertained the idea of reciprocating. So I wasn't *that* surprised when the conversation turned sexual.

Gary: "Sooo . . . what are you wearing?"

Me: (glancing down at the bubbles) ". . . uh, honesty or imagination?"

Did I mention that I didn't have great boundaries in those days, especially with men (remember my ex-boyfriend)? This drunk guy wanted to have phone sex, and I didn't know how to get out of the conversation.

Cue the dread. God, I wish I had some group therapy homework to talk about right now, I thought in a sudsy panic. But I was already in too deep.

My mind froze. The pressure of delivering some kind of hot and sexy verbal performance to become the person I imagined Gary wanted me to be short-circuited my brain. I opened my mouth to say something risqué, but couldn't think of anything that didn't sound fake and cheesy.

Do I go full porno dialogue? "Oh no! I'm all out of money! However will I pay for this pizza?" Absolutely not. It's way too fake, and I'm not a phone-sex operator. He'll know it's not real or think I'm mocking him.

Do I try to be witty about it? "I'm in this bath and I'm so . . . wet." I'm not going to stoop to cheap double entendre puns. It's so dumb it's not even attractive.

Maybe go with a classic? "Is that a banana in my . . . bath?" Wait, no. That doesn't work.

Trying to figure out what to say, I sat up too fast, sloshing water over the side of the tub, and instinctively tried to scoop more bubbles around myself—as if Gary could see me through the phone. I didn't know who to be, what to do, or what to say.

Not knowing what else to do, I just went along with this drunk fool on the other end of the line. *Sarah has mentally left the building.*

In my dissociative stupor, I ran out of ideas. All I could think of was literally the worst choice someone could make while having phone sex. "I want to lay with you . . . Biblically."

Did I just say, "I want to lay with you biblically?" *What is wrong with me? Jesus, take the phone!*

Fourth mistake: don't have phone sex like a goddamn puritan nun.

I immediately considered dropping my phone in the bathwater, which had all at once gone cold. But it was an iPhone, and those aren't cheap. I even thought about faking my own death by "drowning" in my bath. Then I could start my life over in the woods to live hidden among the forest creatures, never to interact with another human ever again. (Based on how things were going so far, I figured I'd fare better with forest animals.)

But I somehow stayed on the line, tossing out awkward half-sentences until it was clear he was too drunk to carry on a meaningful conversation anyway.

Gary: ". . . you still there? Mmm . . . wait, what was I . . ? Never mind. I'm . . . tired."

Me: "Goodnight, Gary." Click.

Thank God he was too drunk to remember what happened—or at least, I can only hope. When he called the next day, his tone was bright, casual, just like usual.

Gary: "Hey, we talked last night, didn't we? What about?"

Me: "Oh, you know. Just . . . stuff."

My pathetic attempt at phone sex is my own little dirty-pure secret.

I hope.

Sleep Over

ACHIRO P. OLWOCH

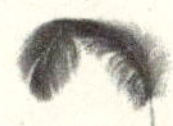

I love sleeping over at Nancy's house. Maybe it's because of the games.

It all starts with us girls showing up at exactly 7:00 pm. Nancy has a rule: anyone who comes in after 7:00 will not be admitted. And there is no such thing as appearing more than five minutes before seven. I know, she is crazy with her rules, but hey, we are the ones who die for her sleepovers. I normally come at least fifteen minutes early and wait in my car. I am not the only one; most of the other girls do the same. Those without cars take *boda bodas,* the ubiquitous (and anonymous) motorcycle taxis, then sit with those of us who drive. It is a weird ritual, but at the end of the day, it is so worth it.

I am a writer, one of the lucky ones who actually

makes a living working as a staff writer for one of the big lifestyle magazines. I never write about any of our girly escapades, though. For good reason. In my little Uganda, we would be arrested and fined for indecency or immorality or something that our minister of ethics would come up with on a whim. That man! I think he needs to attend one of our sleepovers just so that he can loosen up. I do not think he is getting as much sex as he would like. *Yoh!*

Nancy is a married woman with a notorious cheating husband. He has hit on half of the women in Kampala and slept with half of those he has hit on. He comes from a very prominent and wealthy family and is not bad to look at. Then again, I do not know anyone who has money and looks bad. He gives Nancy whatever she wants whenever she wants and, in exchange, she tolerates his two-timing habits. They still share their marital bed, but there is nothing marital about it. No intimacy whatsoever. It is more awkward than a brother and sister sharing a bed. If she accidentally touches him, he cringes like a snake has bitten him, and she prefers that he doesn't touch her either.

After the first year, Nancy made a decision—not out of desperation, but out of clarity. If her husband would not touch her, would not even look at her the way he once did, then she would stop asking. She would stop shrinking. But instead of slipping into a quiet affair, Nancy chose something else entirely. She built something. A space.

Why the parties? Why not just cheat and be done with it?

Because Nancy understood something most people don't say out loud: sex doesn't cure loneliness. It's about being seen. She didn't just want pleasure—she wanted permission to have pleasure. And she wanted to offer that permission to others, too.

She started reaching out to a few women she knew—not out of pity, not out of manipulation, but recognition. Some were also dealing with sexless marriages, others with partners who saw them only in chore lists and dinner plates. Not all of them were unhappy. But all of them were hungry. Not just for touch, but for freedom. For joy. For mischief without guilt. A few of us aren't married at all, but we come because Nancy's parties remind us of something we forget too easily: we're allowed to want more.

With the millions her husband lets her have—and maybe, yes, this is her revenge—Nancy rents a house she visits once a month. Fully furnished, unapologetically lavish. A chef is hired. The lights are low. The music plays softly in the background. And none of us pays a cent.

"Oh! No need to lift a finger," she says. "This is *my* gift to you all. Think of it like a kind of burnt offering to the gods of chaos, a remedy to solve all our intimacy problems. All you're allowed to do is show up and act grateful, like guests at a surprise party."

It all starts with dinner and light chatter as we all catch each other up with what's been going on in our lives over the month. Tonight, there are nine of us. One by one, we disappear from the table and head to one of eight private suites. As we bathe in our private bathrooms, we allow our minds to wander, contemplating who we'd like to end up with. Nancy makes sure that she is the last one at the table, then decides who to visit. She knows we fight like hungry rats to share a bedroom with her.

Tonight, Nancy chooses the bedroom where I'm already tangled up with Jade. The lights are low, golden, humming against the shadows. I'm lying on my back, half-dressed, my lips swollen from kissing Jade, who is hovering above me, her hair a curtain, her breath soft against my cheek.

I like Jade very much. She has this giggle that makes my female parts dance. She's all angles and elegance—long limbs, sharp collar bones—and somehow she always smells like strawberries, like she's just walked through a summer field. For someone so slender, her fingers are thick, steady, grounding; best of all, she knows exactly what to do with them. There's something confident about her touch. Not rushed. Not performative. Just . . . attentive. Like she's listening with her hands.

In the real world, Jade is a lawyer. Wears heels, reads contracts, probably terrifies men in boardrooms. She's still single, and I'm not sure if she calls herself a lesbian. But labels don't matter much in this house. She knows how to make another woman feel worshipped. Did I mention I like Jade? I *really* like her.

I also love the way Nancy enters a room.

She doesn't knock. She doesn't need to. She enters like a shift in the atmosphere. Velvet and thunder. Her presence alone changes the oxygen in the room.

God, her husband doesn't know what he's missing.

Nancy doesn't speak at first. Just walks in slowly, barefoot, silk robe falling open at the throat. She smiles, not like someone asking permission, but like someone who already knows the answer. When she joins us, Jade and I exhale.

Nancy takes what I'm already feeling with Jade and lifts it, stretches it, deepens it, adding harmony to a single note. She doesn't interrupt. She enhances. She turns touch into ritual. Kissing Jade's shoulder. Pressing her palm against my chest. Looking at me like I'm something worth savoring.

With Nancy, everything feels intentional. Curated. She knows how to move, how to wait, how to take her time. And in that moment, I forget whatever life exists outside this house. All I know is the heat of their skin, the smell of strawberries and vanilla, and the way Nancy's voice sounds like a dare when she finally whispers, "Don't stop."

Jade doesn't pause. Her hand keeps moving, firm and steady, pressing through the thin fabric between my legs. Her lips are soft on mine, but there's fire behind the softness. I arch slightly, breath catching.

Nancy moves closer. Her presence alone pulls the temperature of the room tighter. She kneels on the bed, fingertips grazing my hip, then slips her fingers under the waistband of my panties. Jade's mouth is at my throat now, and her hands cup my breasts, and still Nancy's fingers don't stop.

Nancy parts my legs. Gently. Intentionally. And then her mouth—hot, wet—finds my clitoris and she sucks it. I gasp. Loudly. I reach for Jade without thinking, tug her toward me. She's already bare, already ready. She swings her leg over Nancy's body, and I pull her close, burying my mouth between her thighs.

We move in rhythm. Nancy's tongue, Jade's hips, my hands gripping whatever flesh they can find. Everything pulses. The lines between who's touching and who's being touched blur. I stop licking. I can't keep going. It's too much. Nancy's fingers are inside me now, and her mouth is relentless. Jade reads it in my face. "Let go," she whispers, almost laughing.

I do. The release crashes through me. I shudder, eyes shut, fists full of sheets.

Nancy rises slowly, lips glistening, eyes fierce with satisfaction. She turns to Jade. I'm still catching my breath.

They're already deep in it, kissing like no one else exists. And for a moment, I feel the edge of being left out. That ache of wanting. So I reach for Jade, needing to finish what I started.

I slide my hand up the inside of her legs, fingers tracing over her slowly, deliberately. She meets my touch with a soft sound and a tilt of her hips. Nancy, using one arm, gently eases Jade onto her back. Jade spreads her legs wide. An invitation, a command. She's glistening, eager, and so ready.

I move towards her clit, lick my fingers gently, and run them over her body. I circle her clit, then slide two fingers inside her, slowly at first, then deeper. She takes me in easily, her body clenching around the rhythm. Nancy lowers herself to kiss and suck softly on Jade's nipples, moving from one to the other like a secret passed between lips.

Jade's close. I feel it in the way her breath falters, in the tension humming through her. I lower my mouth to her clit, flicking, sucking, while my fingers keep moving in and out of her, faster now. She arches up into me, moaning, hands gripping the sheets.

Nancy leans in, gently brushes my mouth aside, and replaces it with her fingers, first tender, then firmer, circling Jade's clit in that perfect rhythm that sends her spiraling. I pull out just in time to watch her body explode. A sharp cry, a burst of wetness, a moment of absolute release. Nancy kisses Jade as she trembles, wrapping her up like a shield and a secret.

Then there's the pause. The good kind. The soft laughter, the shared breath. Nancy points to a jug of juice on the nightstand. We pour ourselves glasses and sip in silence, letting the moment cool. That's one of the best parts, honestly, the in-between. We reset.

Jade heads to the shower. I follow a few minutes later, craving the water, the warmth, and her skin against mine. We start kissing under the spray. Slow, playful. Nancy joins us, bare and radiant. We offer to help her wash. She grins. The steam rises around us, and we bask in it.

There's loud laughter, moaning from the other bedrooms, the distant hum of music Nancy always makes sure is playing to muffle the sounds. The house is walled, private. Still, I wonder what the neighbors must think. All the smoke, the shouting, the ritualistic weeping at midnight. If they're not calling the police, they're definitely updating the group chat.

For us, it doesn't matter.

Jade and I want Nancy. We both reach for her at once, grinning like girls with a shared secret. She loves to be touched. We know that. I get there first, my fingers slipping into her, and she gasps. Not from surprise, from pleasure. Jade slides in beside me, her hands exploring Nancy's breasts, joining the rhythm.

Nancy braces herself against the shower wall, back arched, legs open. She's moaning now, quietly, almost reverently. My fingers press deeper into her, then shift. I circle behind, slipping one finger in, then two. She lets out a shuddering breath.

Jade has her fingers inside too, moving in tandem. Nancy's body starts to shake in pleasure. She comes in silence, only a long, low sigh escaping her lips. Then she collapses softly into Jade's arms.

The three of us rinse slowly. The water cools us down before we dry off and climb back into bed.

We'll need to rest. Just for a little while. The night isn't done with us yet.

It's customary here—a kind of unspoken rule—that anyone can rotate bedrooms if they want to. It's all about pleasure. Pleasure and more pleasure. So, rotation is encouraged. Celebrated, even.

I don't want to rotate. Not at all. Selfishly, I hope no one tries to come into our room. When it's just Jade and me, we leave the door unlocked, part invitation, part indifference. But once Nancy joins us from the shower, she locks the bedroom door, like she's sealing a vault.

People keep trying the handle. Not knocking. Just casually, like it's a fridge they hope has something better inside this time. You hear the click, the pause, and then the soft shuffle of disappointment as they move on to the next bedroom.

At one point, someone clears their throat dramatically, like maybe the door will take the hint and open itself out of politeness. We try not to laugh, but it's hard not to when your love life has a queue system and zero signage.

We did not make it to another session that night. We just started talking . . . and talking and talking till we fall asleep.

The next morning, we emerge to the smell of bacon and sausages. The chef is back and as we gather back around the table, we all giggle each time we encounter him. I guess he is used to these sleepovers. He is paid as much as if he cooked for the whole month for working one night and morning. His silence is bought, but Nancy made him sign a non-disclosure agreement anyway. We cannot have anyone talking about what goes on here. Not that it is anyone's business anyway. But still. We appreciate that he knows how to keep our secrets.

After breakfast, we begrudgingly head back to our individual routines: pretending, smiling too much, avoiding certain questions, clinging to the glow from the night before. Lipstick smudged, thighs aching, hearts a little lighter. We don't say much. Just long hugs, knowing looks, and promises to meet again. But the truth is: every time we gather, it could be the last.

That's what no one says out loud.

When we're inside the house, we laugh and kiss and touch as if the world outside can't harm us. But it can. We live in a place where what we do is illegal. Where women like us—queer, loud, unapologetically desiring—disappear in headlines or are buried in rumor. Where all it takes is one whisper in the wrong ear.

So yes, we live boldly. But never carelessly.

Every gathering is a gamble. Every orgasm is a middle finger to the law. Every soft moan in the dark is a form of protest. We know this. We feel it when the music dips and the silence creeps in. But we choose joy anyway.

We choose each other. Because one night of freedom is still freedom. And sometimes, that's everything.

Firsts

YIN XZI HO

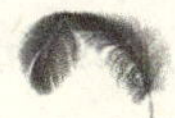

The first time a boy kissed me, I was seventeen and didn't see it coming. It was a there-and-gone thing. Wet and cold and then over. We had been watching an episode of *Futurama*—one of his favorite shows—ruined for me forever by this one, unwanted act.

I turned to him, confused. He looked back, expectant.

"Oh shit, was that your first kiss?"

I nodded.

"Well, I'm sorry it wasn't *perfect*, and I'm sorry it didn't happen at sunset on the beach while dolphins jumped through the sea." A pubescent voice crack undermined the derisiveness of his words, but it cut me all the same.

My inner voice screamed at me to remain calm, to

be unflappable, to not anger and possibly lose the boy I had started to like. I faced the TV again, watching an animated red-haired man-boy shake his fist at a silver robot. The fan above our heads blew against my lips and called attention to the wetness of my mouth until it was the only thing I could think about.

There's no guidebook to your first times, especially when they go bad. All you can do is ask yourself questions. *Is wiping off his saliva rude? Will he take that as a signal that I want another kiss?* I certainly didn't. What I wanted was to shiver so hard I would spontaneously explode into existence somewhere else—my home, the middle of a grocery store, somewhere clean and brightly lit. Anywhere other than this living room lit only by the TV playing a show I could no longer process, next to a boy who had taken my first kiss.

A couple of months later, I had a panic attack when that same boy tried to cajole me into making him come. We'd gotten over the excruciating minefield that was navigating our mouths together, had figured out how to angle our heads so that his nose no longer hit my glasses, had done it enough that I had started to like it. But this? The act of him bringing my hand to his penis, having to navigate through a zipper, and the folds of boxers?

I was so scared, I lost the ability to breathe. Or

maybe I chose to stop breathing so I wouldn't have to keep touching the pale, fleshy thing between his legs that was trying to stand. I'm still not sure which version is true, but when my brain registered the lack of oxygen and kicked my breathing into overdrive to ensure survival, he finally noticed he wasn't going to get his hand job.

As he curled his body around mine, a single, lucid thought rose to the surface of my mind: maybe we can do this—be a thing, I mean. Look at him being nice and supportive. Then the panic attack took over, and my next thought was, This would be a dumb way to die.

I tried to ground myself by opening my eyes, but my tears blurred the sight of his crumpled bedding, spinning it like a washing machine on a rinse cycle. Curled behind me, the boy was saying something, but the sawing of my breathing cut through his words. Eventually, when my tears subsided and the snail trail of snot from my nose to the bed had dried, he rolled me so we were facing each other. With a small smile, he brushed the hair from my face and said, "That was hot."

The first time I had sex, I was twenty. We were both in a foreign country for a semester abroad, which is how we met. This time, I did not have a panic attack upon seeing his penis; this time, I was sure I was in love. Before you get your hopes up, however, let me assure you—this guy did not raise the fucking bar.

Picture this: I am on the bottom, trying desperately to figure out what to do with all of my limbs. *Should my hands clasp his shoulders? What the hell should I be doing with my feet? With my knees?* I'm thinking these thoughts as he's thrusting into me, and then I remember, Yin Xzi, be in the moment! Don't forget to enjoy this! So I smile at him, because smiling is sexy, right? Then he pulls out of me, brings his right hand to his penis, and comes vigorously across my stomach. Before I have time to do *anything* (fake moan, gasp, say "thank you for coming" like a convenience store clerk), he looks at me and says, "I know that was your first time, but it was kind of disappointing."

The night before this disaster, this boy had tried to initiate sex—he, already hard, me, unsure of whether what I was doing was right. Before we had gotten into bed, he'd pulled me close and told me that there was no need to put my pajamas on, that he loved my body as it was. He kissed the side of my neck, and I tried not to shy away. Then we were naked and horizontal in a twin bed. He ducked his head to nuzzle my ear.

"I'm ticklish," I reminded him again, cheeks itching with embarrassment at how childish I sounded.

"Come on," he urged as he thrust his hips at mine. "You know you're into this."

I did not, in fact, know that I was into this, wasn't sure what aspect of it I should be into at all. Even though my breathing was slow and even, my brain decided it was a great time to play the audio clip of my first boyfriend finding my hyperventilation "hot."

Maybe it would work a second time, I thought, and tried to breathe erratically.

"You okay?" he asked, stilling on his forearms to look at me.

"Mhmm," I breathed, still smiling at him. He nodded and began to grind again. I tried to focus on his warm brown eyes, not the hard nudging happening between my legs.

"Okay, well," he said in between kisses. "Let's relax a little, okay?"

His hand crept down between my legs to separate my thighs a little more.

I obliged.

He pushed against me a couple more times, his frustration mounting each time my body wouldn't let him in. It didn't hurt. It felt more like he was knocking on a door; I imagined my pubic bone folding downward like a shield.

"Well, this is clearly not happening tonight," he

groaned, half-heartedly touching himself as he grew limp.

"I'm sorry," I said. I wasn't.

"It's okay," he said, tucking his face into my neck. I tried to remain as I was, splayed across the twin bed, body goose-pimpled and going cold above the blankets as he entwined a warm leg over mine. "We can try again tomorrow."

Now I lay there as he collapsed beside me in the twin-sized bed, thinking about the yellow of the sheets. And the whisper of cracks across the ceiling of his dorm room. The boy wiped off his penis with the T-shirt he'd taken off the night before. Outside, birds chirped faintly, and next to me, the boy started absentmindedly flicking through his phone. Instagram photos of other girls on beach vacations, interspersed with soccer players, scrolled through my periphery.

"You should probably go pee," he said.

"Right," I responded, thinking about seventh-grade sex ed. But the cum cooling on my stomach gave me pause. Even as I watched it rise and fall as I breathed, it felt like a brick sitting on my torso. The air around me grew gelatinous and dense, trapping my body against the yellow sheets.

"Hey," he nudged me. "It's okay, go pee and clean up."

I nodded again and moved my hands through the Jell-O of the air to cup the area under the cum, watching it slide against my skin and onto my fingers as I sat up. I stood up to tiptoe to the bathroom down the hall, intensely grateful that his room was the only one on the floor.

Once in the shower, I braced myself for the slow-to-heat water and aimed my stomach at the waist-high tap. As I peed, I hoped that gravity would be on my side. I tried not to even breathe the word "pregnant," as if a stray thought would manifest as a baby in my uterus.

The worst thing about these firsts isn't how long it took me to come to terms with them or share them with someone else. The worst part is how they have attempted to bury the firsts I have since come to love.

The first time I asked a boy to be in a committed, monogamous relationship with me, it was awkward as hell. We were sitting side by side on a bench in the dark, with a cold wind whipping into our faces and a few pieces of sushi left in the box on my lap.

"So, the reason I ask about past relationships is, well, we haven't talked about it in the course of our friendship and also . . .I think we could be in one, a relationship, I mean, if you want?" I peered intently at the dollop of wasabi in the corner of the to-go box, trying to identify its exact shade of green, trying not to think about the green of the eyes of the boy next to me.

"Yin Xzi," he said, tapping me till I looked at him. His mouth kept moving, and he sounded hesitant, and then there was blood drumming frantically through my head until I realized that he had been saying yes. "Yes, yes, I would. I would like that."

Yes! My body was a series of fireworks. He said yes! I leaned into him, giddy with closeness. His eyes softened as he drew his eyes closer to my face and—*oh no, not this right now.*

"I hate first kisses," I blurted. I should've just shoved my mouth full of sushi instead. No one kisses someone with a mouthful of raw fish. I flinched pre-emptively.

"That's okay. It doesn't have to be now."

"Great!" I shrilled, fiddling with the waxy cardboard. "I just find kissing very weird."

"Can I drive you home?"

I nodded, shaking with relief as I tossed the to-go box in a trash can, my stomach roiling with adrenaline. We chatted about small things like the upcoming weekend's weather and our respective plans for the next day.

When he eased into park on the road in front of my house, the car quieted until I could hear our breathing.

He looked at me.

"Can I kiss you now?"

"No, I . . .I really don't like first kisses."

"Okay, that's okay. What about a goodnight hug?"

We got out of the car, and he pulled me close.

When we finally did kiss, it was on my terms. We were cuddling together in bed, but I was fidgeting more than usual.

"What's up?" he asked, shifting both of us so that we were facing each other.

"You know what I think is really attractive?" I was grateful for the half-dark of my bedroom, but I could still feel his gaze on me. "When, like, someone asks another person for permission to kiss them. I think it's really cute. It's soft. But also confident. And kinda sexy . . ."

My voice died away as I met his eyes.

"Can I kiss you?" His voice was thick with nerves, and tender and warm, and I nodded, heart crawling up my throat. I closed my eyes, and this time, instead of unexpected lips, instead of being stiff, I received a soft kiss. It was phenomenal.

Pineapples in the Snow

KATE HESKETT

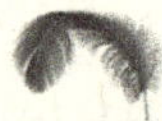

At thirty-five years old, when it came to my sexuality, I had more questions than answers.

I'd managed to find myself a Canadian boyfriend before Covid hit, and we'd buckled down to weather the storm together, living for free in the house his father built back in the 80s. I came out of the pandemic with a common-law relationship, a permanent residency card, and a beautiful black Covid-cat. But having lost a few years to social isolation, I also emerged with a renewed commitment to pursuing the exciting love life I'd always wanted.

The problem was I'd landed in yet another long-term domestic partnership, with a man I loved dearly but who, ultimately, and despite initially being on board, could not reconcile his love for me with my love for many.

I tried to explain it. I sent him articles. I read books. I joined Facebook support groups. But no amount of friendship or food analogies could shift his belief that love is a zero-sum game. Despite his own non-monogamous fantasies (who doesn't want a threesome?), when the world opened up, my partner decided he could not. I felt stuck, angry and resentful, and also incredibly guilty, as I watched the person I loved pull away from me and lean into worsening drug addiction. It was the worst of both worlds, and although I was faithful to him, I felt like I was cheating on myself.

But what if being open didn't suit me at all? I'd never actually been in a non-monogamous relationship. What if I was blowing up my home life for some kind of grass-is-greener fantasy? After a lifetime of questioning the "rules" of relationships, I was convinced the only way to know for sure was to try. When a friend recommended buying a solo ticket to a three-day swingers' hotel takeover in the fall, I was listening.

Unable to work while I waited for my permanent residency, I had very few friends in Whistler. With no budget to spend on swimwear, I took to swimming naked at Lost Lake's clothing-optional dock and was stoked to uncover a small community of very friendly and politely pervy people.

Over two summers, this collection of mostly older men became my entire social circle, which is how I found myself naked and drip-drying, complaining about my non-existent sex life to a very fit, tanned, and much older Whistler local.

"It's right in the village. Super expensive to get a room, but you can get a ticket just to the event and go home to sleep in your own bed at night. I wish I could go, but we're doing one of their cruises in December."

"I thought you had to be a couple to be a swinger?"

"Not at the big parties. Swingers love a single lady," he says, giving me a side-eye and a double eyebrow raise.

I groan, "Not a lady, remember?"

"I know, but . . ." he lowers his shades and looks directly at my naked breasts, ". . . with those boobs you could get all the dick and pussy you want."

I roll my eyes and push my cleavage together.

"Yeah? With these?"

The poor man practically salivated. It was a cheap trick to regain the upper hand in our flirtation, but it worked. And as much as I complain about having to continuously wrangle them into submission, I knew he was right. My boobs have always been a handy shortcut to getting laid.

At the time, it seemed like a gentler way to open up

my relationship, as I wouldn't be actively dating or seeking out a particular person or romance. Ideally, there would have been some kind of meet-and-greet nearby, where I could've socialized with like-minded people over a casual drink or two. But with no visible queer, let alone polyamorous, community available to me in Whistler, my first toe-dip into the lifestyle culture was more like hurtling myself headfirst down a skeleton track.

I'd attended a very structured (and kinky) sensuality workshop and play-space a few years earlier in Melbourne, my hometown, but hadn't been able to find anything in the realm of pleasure and exploration since relocating to Canada. And like my sex life in general, it was something I'd mostly given up on in exchange for safety. Safety from the plague, but also safety from losing my relationship and my housing.

When I got home, I looked up the company my friend recommended, and sure enough, there was a large, legit swingers' party coming to town. The website was loaded with information about security, sexual safety, and consent culture, as well as party themes, icebreaker games, and a schedule of daily sexuality and wellness workshops. It wasn't cheap, costing about as much as half a season's ski pass, but I told myself that, even if all I did was go to a few daytime sessions and hang out in the hot tub, it would be a worthwhile experience. What did I have to lose? I desperately needed to get out of my ill-fitting monogamous shell, allow some creative energy to flow, and tend to the parts of myself I'd had to tuck away like the corners of ill-fitting bedsheets.

As for my partner, I told him that I didn't know anyone who was going, that even though it was in Whistler, almost everybody was coming from out of town. I tried to convince him to come with me, to see first-hand what it might be like to love differently.

Weeks passed with no response. Eventually, I asked for a hall pass, a permission slip to take a sanctioned absence from the relationship restraints I was tangled in.

I bought my ticket.

As the event drew closer, I tried my best to put on an everything-is-normal face for my partner, but my excitement and anxiety left me buzzing with what-ifs. Not only was I risking a long-term relationship I'd already put a fuck-tonne of effort into, but I was going to show up to an event with two hundred plus scantily clad strangers *by myself*. I didn't know what to expect, I didn't know what to wear, and most of all, I didn't know what gender to show up as.

Days at the lake were getting shorter, the September

sun no longer strong enough to dry off without a towel. With limited dock days left, and no one else to talk to, I reluctantly lowered my body-positive mask and asked my friend if I'd be expected to look a certain way, as I'd read online that some spaces had expectations around "personal maintenance."

"Like showering?"

"Nooo." I clenched my fists open and closed. "Like for women, like makeup, and nails, and now it seems—" I took a deep breath and gestured to his bald junk, "everybody is expected to be hairless."

There it was. The elephant, not in the bush, but rather swinging freely between his legs.

"And I . . ." I air-palmed my furry body—my luscious underarm hair, my curly bush poking out from beneath my tummy rolls, my downy legs—". . . am not."

I frowned at my rainbow-painted toes. This was not a conversation I'd been planning to have with a sixty-something straight man. But somehow it seemed more natural to talk about my body hair with someone who was already looking at it.

We'd had the "not a woman" talk before, but given we only ever met naked, without any gender-coded clothes on, the dock had become an unexpected gender-free hideout for me and my fat, hairy body. Like I was simply part of the 60s hippy ski-bum scene, and not a 21st-century closeted poly-bi-enby. Maybe what I really needed was some kind of nudist swingers party? A version of *Dating Naked,* but for non-monogamous, pangender folx?

"What if I show up and there's no one else who looks like me?"

My friend nodded. "You should just go as yourself," he said, "however you feel comfortable."

I raised my eyes to his, looking for any signs of facetiousness, but found none. A slow smile spread across his face.

"The right people will find you."

When the night I've spent so long imagining finally arrives, I am in near panic. Despite my friend's advice, I've decided I'll feel safest if I "performed woman" for the weekend and paid an aesthetician to make me look compliant. I'd even gone and bought makeup for the first time in a decade, including waterproof mascara for the hot tub and a slut-red lip color for the slutting.

As the dress-up theme for the welcome soiree is Reggae Beach, I'd dug out an old blue bikini with palm fronds, my Australian Havaiana thongs with the diamanté detail, and an orange and green sarong I'd legitimately bought in Bali. Comfy enough, but not really appropriate attire for commuting through the early November snow. I don't want to walk to the hotel, but I also don't want to ask my partner for a lift, preferring to at least keep the illusion of a normal night out, for both our sakes.

If I don't do this now, though, I worry I never will. Because as much as I push back against all the people who said I can't have love *and* freedom—my friends, my family, my exes—the lifetime of evidence I've acquired so far says that they are right.

Having waited too long to call for a cab, I ask my father-in-law/landlord/housemate for a lift. The request for transportation is not unusual, but I can tell he is curious about the beachwear, the location, my bright red lips, and dark eyes. So when we pull up at the Whistler Inn and Suites, and a woman runs past in a sequined bikini, I grab my hiking pack of supplies and jump out of the car with a hasty, "I'll taxi home!" and, in case he is watching, walk into the foyer with my head held high.

My first stop is the check-in table, where I sign the Rules of Play and get wrist-banded. Most of the rules apply to any hotel stay—*please clean up after yourself, no glass in the pool area*—but I am amused to see "fraternizing with staff is prohibited" and the universal safeword for the weekend is "Meatloaf." At the welcome table, I make myself a bead name necklace and bedazzle my free tumbler with some jewels, a flamingo, and a giant googly eye. Some people are doing some intricate design work, but I haven't come here to play arts and crafts.

I drop my daypack at the designated ski lockers and open one of the gin cans I've brought with me. After much deliberation at the liquor store and many warnings from the organizer about not overdoing the alcohol, I had decided to go with my on-mountain ski-pocket favorite, the Black Fly Gin Fizz. Not only does the pretty pink can with the splattered black fly match the snowboarding pants at home in my closet, the low-carbonated grapefruit juice still tastes good at body temperature after being carried around all day.

As prepared as I can be, I take a deep breath and open the door to the welcome soiree, only to be slammed with a wall of heat and noise.

The small room is completely packed with sweaty, semi-naked people, all yelling to be heard over the extremely loud DJ in the corner. Some folks are managing to have conversations, but their heads are pressed so close together I can't imagine casually joining in. I stand with my back flat against the wall and pretend to wait for someone while I gulp my gin fizz. Sweat drips down my brow, and I am thankful I'd invested in waterproof mascara. This is not my scene. I escape back to my locker, grab some extra cans, and go in search of the hot tub.

To my surprise, I am not the only one keen to leave the party early, because there are already a handful of people soaking up the steamy quiet. Some of them are even naked! Which means I can hot tub and keep my costume bikini dry.

As I peel off my swimming outfit, I notice a curvaceous vision with long red-brown hair lounging on the edge of the tub in a pin-up style, crimson one-piece. She smiles and holds out a Tupperware container of homemade, pineapple-shaped sugar cookies. "Want some? I've eaten too many."

"They're so good," says her partner, reaching for another. He doesn't look like he eats a lot of cookies. He has a lean, muscular frame, a narrow waist, and a beard that's grown in just enough not to be scratchy.

Regulars at the annual hotel takeover—they call it sexy summer camp—committed couple Amy and Zack are also hiding from the noise and the overwhelm. We bond quickly over drinking the same pink gin cans and a need for quiet corners. Zack and I also share a love of Aussie hip-hop, and we chat about Butterfingers and The Herd and Hilltop Hoods.

"I love the lack of ego. And the humor," I say.

"No 'bitch this, bitch that.'"

"Have you heard 'Dear Science' by Seth Sentry?"

"Don't think so."

"It's a whole song complaining about a lack of hoverboards." I sing a few lines, much to his amusement.

"So do you watch MasterChef Australia?" Zack asks.

I laugh, not reading the room. "God, no. I mean the first season, yes, when it was new and we didn't know the formula yet, but otherwise—"

"We've seen every episode," he says, cerulean eyes now wary.

"Every episode?"

"Of every season."

I look to Amy for some indication that he's joking. "Even the old ones?"

Amy is sucking on the straw in her pineapple tumbler cup. She nods enthusiastically. Removing the straw from her lips, she adds, "It's our date night go-to. If Zack's away for work, I'm not allowed to watch it until he gets back." She pouts.

I am quite tipsy, but she looks genuinely aggrieved. I do my best to atone. "It is quite popular back home, a lot of people like it," I say. "But isn't there a Canadian one?"

"Yeah, but it sucks," Zack says. "The Australians

are just so nice to each other, and it's a really supportive environment. They all help each other out. And it's more about the food than the competition. We love food. Amy, you need to drink water."

I turn my head and see Amy lying on the edge of the hot tub, her cheek resting on her hands, her colorful eyelids closed.

"But I'm so sleepy," she says, sounding half asleep already.

Zack gets out of the tub and starts gathering her things.

"I have to take Amy to bed."

I nod, trying to hide my disappointment. "Of course, no worries."

I'd been enjoying our conversation, the quick sparks and following each other's tangents. Two minds playing together in the sandpit. But it's only the first night, and Amy really isn't going to last.

"How long do you think you'll stay? Will you be here if I come back?" he asks.

Possibility flutters in my stomach. Does that mean what I think it means?

"Yes? I'll be here."

"Okay, I'll see you in a bit."

He flashes me a hungry smile, wraps Amy in a white robe, and is gone.

While I wait for Zack, I strike up a conversation with a couple from Squamish. He asks for permission to touch me, and though I'm mildly disappointed when his wife declares she's "strictly dick," his gentle stroking more than makes up for it. I find myself feeling very relaxed, the hot water soothing away all the stress I went through to get here. I lean back against the tub and close my eyes, enjoying the light pressure applied right where I need it. This man I just met knows how to make me feel good. So good that my mouth opens wide and I suck in air sharply, becoming suddenly aware that I have an audience.

Strictly Dick pushes her tongue against the inside of her cheek. "He's good with his fingers, isn't he?" She looks . . . horny. Did watching her partner make me come turn her on?

Sitting on the other side of the hot tub, Zack is staring at me intently. Shit! I didn't know he was back. He saw that? I close my eyes and try to hide in plain sight. I've probably blown it now. He'll think I'm not interested in him. Or that I'm easy. Or spoiled goods. Or . . .

When I summon up the courage to open my eyes and look at Zack's face, he's grinning, eyes wide with excitement. This is not the look of someone who is turned off.

I end my interaction with the man, muttering something like "Thank you for your service," and cross the tub to sit next to Zack.

"Hi," I manage, looking sheepish.

"Hi!"

"I didn't notice you'd come back."

"No," he says, "you were busy." He chuckles and opens his legs to let his knee touch mine. As we pick up our conversation, I stroke his calf with the top of my foot. Through the water, I can see the effect my body is having on his.

"Can I kiss you?" he asks.

His lips are soft, his tongue playful. We disappear into each other, a deep and searching make-out session, cut short when Strictly Dick convinces someone to fuck her in the hot tub. Curious, we both turn to watch.

"Isn't the hot tub a no-sex zone?" I ask.

"Yep."

"It seems . . . unhygienic."

Everyone in the tub signed the Rules of Play, but no one tells the fuckers to stop. Ironically, the actual sex kills our sexy mood. Zack looks as grossed out as I am. "Do you want to move to a playroom?" he says.

Many hours later, we exit the playroom, sleepy-eyed and satisfied. Having burned all our cookie energy getting to know each other's bodies, Zack goes back to his bed and Amy, while I return to the ski lockers to change into my warm gear and snow boots. Walking home, I try to process the night's events. As I fall asleep, I can hear my partner snoring in the other room, but all I can think about are the possibilities for tomorrow.

I sleep late into the day and wake to an empty house, thankful for the sanctuary and the quiet. There are no "good morning" messages from my partner, which is disappointing but probably for the best. I don't know what to say to him.

To make the most of my ticket, I've pre-registered for a Learn to Lap Dance class this afternoon. The description sounds inclusive: "bring a partner or come alone" to learn "masculine energy moves." It says we'll be using a chair to "excite and entice." The chair has the added benefit of providing a place to rest when needed and gives participants the option of performing the whole routine sitting, making it a fun time for "all bodies." So, despite my feminist skepticism and my hangover, I drag my butt out of bed, cram my pack full of everything I'll need for Day Two, and hike back to the hotel.

The class is much better than I expected. I love watching a very attractive but not particularly coordinated man learn the routine for his female partner, proving the instructor's point that it's more about attitude than technique. And I'm surprised to learn that when the instructor says, "Now just move in a way that makes you feel sexy in your body," most people know what to do.

I have no clue what to do, and spend several minutes trying to remember a time when I felt sexy in my body.

I can't.

Do other people feel sexy in their bodies? It's a question I'm still pondering as I use the washroom at the pool to get dressed and made-up for the glow party at Garf's. Making my way underground to the local nightclub, the steep stairs and sticky carpet feel familiar. But inside, the black lights and rave-wear can't hide the fact that this is a very different crowd from the local scene.

For starters, the average age has risen about thirty years, judging by the moves on the dance floor. I don't recognize anyone and my sorry excuse for a costume—a thin, low-cut white T-shirt with a black cotton mini-skirt and black pleather boots—looks shitty compared to the plethora of neon fishnets, rainbow faux-fur animal add-ons, and sparkling tittie-tassels. Looking around, I can't see Zack and Amy anywhere. I sidle up to the bar and cash in my two drink tickets for a double gin and tonic.

I've been thinking about Zack all day, fantasizing

about the possibility of some more time together. But I'm also worried. I asked Zack about his relationship rules before we hooked up, not wanting to cause any issues or be seen as some kind of homewrecker. He told me they were both free to play separately, and that Amy would be fine with it. But is it really okay? Or am I about to be outcast for overstepping lines I couldn't see?

Moving back through the crowd with my drink, I see Amy tottering toward me in white platform knee-highs, Zack trailing behind.

"Kaaaaaaaaaaaayyyyyte!"

When she throws her arms around me in a big hello hug, it doesn't feel real.

"Where have you been all day?"

Wait, did she miss me? "Uh, at home? And then at the pool? I didn't get to bed until about five."

"Zack was up really late as well. He's not usually up past midnight."

She shoots Zack a look, and he shrugs and bats his eyelids, feigning innocence.

Does she know he was with me? I try to catch his eye, but he's looking around the room like he needs an escape. My heart thumps louder than the music. Maybe he wants me to leave?

"Do you know where the washrooms are?" Amy asks.

I point her towards the back of the club, past the oversized wooden saloon chair where two women are making out.

"I was hoping I'd see you today," I say to Zack.

"Yeah?" He flashes a smile. "You don't seem excited."

"Sorry, I just . . ." I open and close my fists a few times, trying to collect my thoughts. I don't want this to be a secret. I'm done hiding. "Does Amy know you were with me last night?" I look up at the disco ball; spears of light pierce the dark and stab into the backs of my eyes. I scrunch them up against the unexpected pain.

"Of course," Zack says, "I told her as soon as I got back to the room." He places a hand gently on my shoulder. "Did you think I wouldn't?"

Amy comes bounding towards us. "Those washrooms are revolting," she puckers her face in disgust. "Let's go back to our room so I can pee. Are you coming with us, Kate?"

When we change into our lingerie costumes, Amy looks in horror at the large greenish-purple bruises on my chest. "Was that Zack?"

I bite my lip and nod.

"You brute!" She throws my T-shirt in his face.

"Not intentional!"

Amy narrows her eyes at him.

"But very satisfying."

I giggle, and Amy rolls her eyes at us. "I bet," she says.

"Can you do my eyeshadow like yours?" I ask. "It's so pretty, and I have no idea what I'm doing; I never wear make-up."

Amy paints my face for me, and the three of us spend the rest of the weekend hanging out together platonically. They show me the mini-dungeon and the sensory play space, and introduce me to all their friends. After seeing the cold ski locker area, they insist that I move my things into their room and give me my own keycard so that I can go in whenever I need to, for costume changes or just to hide away and chill out.

On the last night of the takeover, I return to Zack and Amy's room to find the lights off and a coffee filter stuck to the closed door, inked with a note.

"Kate—Come, stay if you like. ~Zack and Amy."

Of all the people who wanted to get to know them better, I'm the one invited in, it's my name on the door.

I swipe my card, excited to play with my friends, but when I open the door, I see that they're cuddled up, fast asleep in their bed. They look so cute, wrapped in each other's arms.

I haven't seen or spoken to my partner in days, and

suddenly feeling very tired, I crawl into the second bed and wrap myself in the soft duvet and drift off to the sound of Amy's light snoring.

When I wake up, Zack and Amy are quietly packing massive amounts of decorations and costumes into designated heavy-duty plastic tubs. When they're done, we stand in the falling snow next to their car and stick our tongues out, trying to catch the flakes before they hit the ground and disappear. They offer to drive me home, and I accept, making sure we hug goodbye before getting in the car.

When they drop me off, Amy has tears. "You'll have to come visit us."

After a lifetime of being shamed and shunned for having feelings for people who were already in relationships, even when I had no intention of disrupting those relationships, I feel like I finally found people who see the world the way I do. Who value relationships with more than one person. For the first time in my life, I think maybe, just maybe, I'm not alone.

Watching them drive away, I can't breathe. I stand at my front door, gasping at the icy air, unable to go inside. I need a hug, but it will take my partner a few weeks to offer me one. I pull out my phone to respond to the only message I received over the weekend.

From my friend at the dock: How's the takeover going? You getting any? Wish I was there.

I wish he was, too. I have so many new stories to tell. But they'll have to wait.

You were right, I reply. I found my people.

Sex Education

ANDREA ANDRES

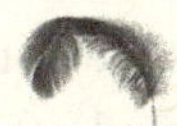

It was two nights before my wedding day.

"Mom, this is going to be *so* special. Just you and me."

"Andrea, I'm so proud to be your mom," she said, giving me a tight squeeze. "I can't believe I have you all to myself tonight!"

"Yup! You do, Mommy Babes," I said, returning her hug.

Mom patted my head as if I were still a little girl. "You'll always be my Annie Babes."

"Mom, I was wondering . . ." My voice trailed off slightly. We were getting ready for bed, and I wanted to ask all my important questions before we fell asleep. As an evangelical pastor's daughter raised in Iowa, our discussion of sex had so far consisted of "wait until marriage." And since they'd opted me out of my school's sex education class, most of what I knew came from a Dr. Dobson curriculum that I followed along with a cassette. It taught me how to be in control of my thoughts and body, what type of woman was pleasing to God, and not to let a boy "go too far."

I was proud that neither my soon-to-be husband nor I had ever gone all the way.

"Mom," I repeated as we got into bed.

"Yeah, hon?" She turned off the light even though, a night owl like me, she did not sound tired.

"You and Dad have been married so long. What's your secret?"

"Never deny your husband," she said with strong conviction.

"Oh?" I didn't doubt her, but I needed more than that. "What do you mean?"

"If your husband wants sex, never say no," she said matter-of-factly. "Men want it more than we do. They need it. It's just biology and the wonderful way God made them."

From our first time, on our wedding night, sex became a job to me. And I could tell that my husband knew it. Over and over. No matter how I talked, what kind of lingerie I wore, or noises I made myself make, I knew I was doing my job poorly. He felt rejected. I told myself and my friend that maybe we didn't have chemistry.

After five years, we started having children, and, as every young mother knows, having young children is exhausting. By the end of each day, I had nothing left to give to anyone. And yet, we had what looked like the perfect marriage: perfect house, perfect kids, perfect bodies, perfect friends. A perfect, active life. But perfect sex? Hmmm.

"Who's going to put the kids to bed?" I asked one evening as I walked into our bathroom. It was larger than the bedroom I'd had growing up.

"Rock, paper, scissors?" he said, grinning. He knew I always won.

"Sure," I said, putting out my hand.

"Rock, paper, scissors," we both chanted.

"Shoot!" he said when my scissors cut his paper.

"Gotcha again," I said and reached for my toothbrush.

"Well, maybe you'll have energy left over for us then?" he said and came in for a kiss.

So, while my body screamed *No!* I searched for a sexy outfit I'd bought recently, after reading yet another Christian book about having sex more often. While my husband tucked in the kids, I put on a necklace, a pair of black lace thong underwear, bright red lipstick, and dark eyeliner. Like a gift waiting to be unwrapped, I flipped my long blond hair over my shoulder and waited on the bed with the sheets just right, silencing the screaming in my head by telling myself, It'll be nice to be in his arms.

I only confided in my journal and a close friend, who was praying for me. I knew I needed help to want him more sexually.

"You're gorgeous," my husband said after coming into the bedroom and quickly closing the door. "Can we do 69?" he asked sheepishly.

"Umm . . . you know we don't do that." I cringe. "We talked about it, remember?"

"Man, your high school boyfriend ruined it for me," he said.

"It's not his fault. I don't like it. It has nothing to do with him. I actually could orgasm that way."

"Then why don't you want it?" he cried. "I wish you liked me. I mean my . . . I like your . . ." Trailing off, he sighed after seeing my disgusted face, "Okay, but can you ride me tonight?"

"Fine," I said, relieved that our business negotiations were over, but after a few minutes of that going nowhere, we did it the same way we always did, missionary style. When he was done, he rolled over, satisfied. I got up, cleaned up in the bathroom, and returned to bed, relieved that my job was done. At least for tonight.

Over the years, we tried everything to get me interested in sexual things, but to no avail. I consistently approached sex with revulsion but persevered in order to keep my husband interested in me and not—as Dr. Dobson and other evangelical preachers and teachers taught me to fear—other women. Or, worst of all, in pornography (which would end up being mostly my fault and not my husband's).

Years later, when I was forty and my husband was forty-five, we deconstructed our faith and came to understand the trauma these and other religious teachings caused us both. We learned about the history of swear words, and then moved on to a British comedy-drama Netflix series called *Sex Education* after our teenage daughter suggested it.

I enjoyed the characters, but there were so many scenes that made my stomach churn. I closed my eyes a lot, but my husband loved it. He was flourishing in the process of validating his sexual identity. Neither of us understood why letting go of our shame-filled past didn't do the same thing for me. Determined to fix this part about myself, I continued watching.

On June 29, 2021, we were into Season Two, Episode Four, in which a young girl bursts into the sex therapist's office and blurts out, "I don't want to have sex." The sex therapist (played by Gillian Anderson) replied without hesitating, "Okay. Not having sex is a valid choice." I froze, transfixed. The young girl clarified. "I don't want to have sex at all. I think I might be broken." OMG, I resonated with that! I always felt broken. Gillian then asked her, "Why don't you start out by telling me how you feel when you think about having sex?" After the young girl explains her lack of connection, Gillian asks her if she knows what asexuality is, explaining, "It's when someone doesn't have any sexual attraction to any sex or gender." The girl says she still wants to fall in love. Gillian says, "Some asexual people still want romantic relationships, but they don't want the sex bit."

I gasped. I heard my husband say, "Shit" under his breath.

Then Gillian said something that sent my body floating off onto the poofiest of clouds, "Sex doesn't make us whole, and so, how could you ever be broken?" My skin crawled with goosebumps, and my bones felt no resistance for the first time in my life. We paused the show. I whispered, "That's me." Neither of us had heard the term asexual before. We tried talking about it, but couldn't. I shed a few tears, and we agreed to give each other some space.

That night, I lay in bed thinking about my mother's advice to never deny my husband sex. I rolled my eyes at the irony of telling that to an asexual. How could she have known? I felt bad for her. Did she feel her job was to serve my dad? What about her? Could never having sex be a possibility for me? I never heard anyone talk about a woman's pleasure. My husband tried to give it to me, but I seemed to get more turned on by watching cottonwood float in the sunlight. I'm so weird, I thought.

I had so much to sift through that I took a few days to process my new identity. Since I no longer denied myself or asked God what to do, I gave myself permission to ask what I wanted. I ran through every scenario in my head. What does Andrea want? OMG, what a concept! Is that allowed? Who knew not wanting sex could be normal? When we first met, my husband suppressed that part of him so much that our energies matched. But now? Ha! We couldn't be more opposite. Our marriage is fucked, because we're not fucking. LOL.

We usually shared everything and valued gaining understanding of how our new perspectives were changing us, but it didn't happen easily this time. I had never felt more alone. We tried to talk about the book I had been reading (*Ace* by Angela Chen) and the

Asexual Visibility and Education Network (AVEN) I had discovered online. Neither helped us move forward. By the fourth day of not talking, I could no longer tolerate the disconnection. The chasm between the pain from our past and the desire to move forward together grew as large as the Grand Canyon. Would we remain married? The unspoken question loomed between us. I knew this conversation was going to be tricky and suggested we could go for a car ride to talk.

As we climbed into our blue Camaro, I could tell he was scared. The sunny day couldn't erase the misery of years spent trying to "fix" me, but I still hoped for the best.

I took a deep breath. "I'm actually learning to validate myself for the first time," I told him, hoping he'd see this, at least, as a positive.

"Are you ever going to want sex with me again?" was all he asked, clearly dejected.

I gathered more of my thoughts before continuing. "Do you remember when you told me the secret you'd never told anyone else? Do you remember how connected you felt to me that day?"

He nodded, and I went on. "And then we had sex, and it was emotionally healing for you? Well, if I want to be interested, I have to emotionally connect that deeply every time I have sex. It's exhausting."

He barely lifted his head, but I could tell something clicked.

So, taking a deep breath, I bravely added, "I know it won't be possible for you to understand this fully. Just like I'll never understand how you see things sexually. But please know I love you."

My husband was always listening and supportive, but he was hurt and, at that moment, it felt like a lost cause.

"What makes this time any different?" he said as we drove Highway 99 towards Whistler. "Why do you feel like you're okay with sex now?"

The radio filled the silence. Alanis Morissette asking, ". . . isn't it ironic, don't ya think?"

"Not that song!" I cried out. "Turn it off."

He agreed with a laugh, pulling over. "A little too ironic. I only wanted to get married to have sex, and I married an asexual."

"I'm sorry—for both of us," was all I could say. I took his hand and looked him in the eye for the first time. "Rob, you're my dearest friend. I don't ever want us to be apart. I tried to imagine us in a polyamory relationship or getting divorced, and that hurt too much. I can't imagine my life without you. And when I dwell on all that, it makes me open to being with you in that way again, even if I'm not interested in sexual things. But if I say no to having sex sometimes, please don't take it personally."

He nodded. "Okay. I know you never think about sexual stuff. When we watched that show, I thought we were done. That upset me a lot. I thought you finally got the excuse you were looking for to never have sex with me again."

"I'm so sorry for all you went through. I don't want to leave you. We've been through so much together."

We hugged and shed a few tears.

As we drove home, Whitney Houston's voice came through the speakers, "I wanna feel the heat with somebody . . ." I recalled my eighth-grade self singing her guts out to that song. It made me realize that I needed to learn how to love myself, including accepting the fact that I might never feel the "heat" for somebody. I promised myself to never pretend in the bedroom ever again.

We drove home and made love in the shed. It was a beautiful, unifying moment. I kept my eyes closed and tried to focus my brain on what I liked about it. I was happy that I could feel okay with giving him head because I knew how much it meant to him. I didn't have to pretend to like it. I just did it nice and slow.

Shortly after, my husband bought me a vibrator, and I have to say that really helped my body respond to pleasure. Thankfully, going after my own pleasure turns him on, too. We also found that a blindfold, along with a bit of indica (weed) or whiskey, are just what I need to help me relax.

I may not think about sexual things as I go about my day, the way my husband does, and other people do. But I came back to sex feeling like I own my own body, and that my pleasure matters as much as my husband's. It's not always easy, but we are figuring it out together.

A few years later, my daughter sat across from me at our small circular table. "Mom, you've come so far," she said in a serious adult tone.

Laughing, I replied, "I couldn't agree more. I feel like you always knew something wasn't quite right."

She nodded.

"Sometimes I still feel twelve inside. How do I have a teenage daughter?"

"Ha ha, Mom." She waved me off, laughing.

"I wish my parents had encouraged me to trust myself and validate my own sexual ethos. We're trying to do that for you and your brother."

"Right on time," was her response. "Remember when you used to make me change clothes if I was showing bra straps, or shamed me for listening to sex podcasts?"

That's when I understood. While my husband and

I wrestled with our faith and explored our sexuality together, our kids were watching us and drawing their own conclusions.

The advice I give my daughter now is nothing like the advice my mom gave me. "Learn what you like and enjoy each other," I tell her. "And if you're both into it, you just go ahead and fuck your brains out, honey."

No Man's Land

PIERRE-OLIVIER GAUDREAULT

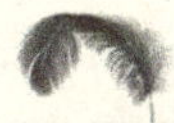

It's spring 2017. I have a large ground-floor apartment in the heart of downtown Montreal—a sublime community on rue Sanguinet, a stone's throw from rue Saint-Denis, in the heart of Quartier Latin—and I'm about to welcome my new roommate, Sébastien.

I've always had an instinct for choosing the right people. Some of my best friends are former roommates, and neighbors hire (read: beg) me to create their ads and meet potential candidates on their behalf.

Sébastien, a Frenchman in his early twenties, is no exception. We first met over a video call, when he explained that he was leaving everything behind—his family, his job, his girlfriend—to try his luck in Montreal. "After my recent break-up and getting laid off, it was time for me to expand my horizons and start something new. I see a bigger life for myself even if that means living far away from my family and friends," he said. I've always found the French more open about what they think and feel, a cultural trait that seems less common on this side of the Atlantic.

I could relate. When I moved to Montreal from the remote countryside of Lac-Saint-Jean a few years earlier, I too left behind my family, my friends, and an ex-boyfriend who reluctantly agreed to try long distance. Despite being in the same province, Montreal had felt like an entirely new world.

A new person in my home will be another new beginning, a change of dynamic. Sébastien turns out to be as charming and charismatic in person as he was on video, and there's something natural and easy about the two of us. We soon start chatting about our respective lives over an evening glass of wine, generally the cabernet sauvignon Ménage à Trois (very fitting, and not on purpose), or the sweet dessert wine Premières Grives from Domaine du Tariquet.

The evenings flow into one another. We quickly move beyond superficial conversations about cultural differences between the French and Québécois to deeper topics that make us vulnerable with one another. I learn that Sébastien always speaks with his heart. As I get to know him, I'm charmed by his *joie de vivre* and inquisitive mind, a little less by his messiness.

I really want our house share arrangement to work, but for me, our place has to look perfect the next day, like something out of a magazine. Cleaning is a coping mechanism that keeps the chaos of my ADHD brain under control. I simply can't help it, but I don't want Sébastien to think I'm crazy. So the minute he leaves, I am down on my knees on the kitchen floor, and not for the fantasy you may imagine. I am scrubbing the greasy floor and washing countertops littered with breadcrumbs and flour after his careless antics in the kitchen, a consequence of his own ADHD. I pray he doesn't walk in and catch me. To be honest, we're actually a lot alike, even though we're also opposites.

A few weeks after he moves in, I get up and wash my wine glass before getting ready for bed; Sébastien does the same. In the hallway leading to our respective bedrooms, I feel his gaze. Is this the work of my fertile imagination? There's a pause, a silence, a palpable tension before he pushes me up against the wall and kisses me.

Well, that's a pleasant surprise.

"Oh my God, your beard," he says as my facial hair brushes his cheeks. His expression is a mixture of surprise and confusion. "You are the first man I've kissed," he admits timidly.

I guess my instinct for choosing roommates has

nothing to do with gaydar, I think to myself, secretly ashamed of my naivety. My mind spins, trying to catch up.

It's wonderful to witness Sébastien's reactions. He seems both overwhelmed and exhilarated. I try to adapt to his rhythm. What's happening feels so right. I can't think straight (get it?) and let myself be carried away by the fire of the moment. My heart begins pounding faster and harder as I feel Sébastien's ardor. It's as if time and space cease to exist; so does my self-control. Events unspool like a movie.

"Your room or mine?" asks Sébastien.

Hello, romantic comedy!

"I don't think going to our bedrooms is a good idea," I reply, momentarily panicked. To me, bedrooms are a clear no man's land for roommates. When living spaces are shared, privacy becomes highly prized and jealously guarded. This is new territory, and I'm anxious to draw a line.

Misère! We know the what and how of the next part of the story, but not the where. With an ever-increasing urgency in our lower bellies, I drag Sébastien to the bathroom. After a brief moment of foreplay on the lid of the toilet seat, we lie on the bathroom floor. I'm oblivious to the cold of the tile, but take a moment to appreciate my Mister Clean tendencies. When my friends say they could eat off my floors, I doubt this is what they have in mind. After the bathroom improvisation that first night, I suggest we upgrade to the living room.

In the weeks that follow, our love affair intensifies, with the couch making the experience less raw. We disappear into the darkness, where nothing exists but one another. We explore, and Sébastien becomes more comfortable. "Oh, I see that you are taking the lead now," I tell him, pleased.

One night, just as I turn Sébastien over to climb onto him, I open my eyes and see a man, a stranger, his nose pressed up against the living room window.

The fire of passion is doused as effectively as a cold shower. "Who the fuck is that?" Sébastien says, clutching a couch cushion to his penis. His reaction reminds me that he has just opened a new door to his sexuality.

"Just a passer-by. Don't worry, he'll go away," I reply as calmly as I can. Sébastien appears to be literally frozen.

But our intruder does not go away. Realizing that he has been spotted, he moves away from the window and starts ringing the doorbell.

My heart pounds for a whole new reason as my eyes fly to the lock. Thank God I didn't forget that in addition to the curtains. "Let's retreat to the hallway," I instruct Sébastien.

We don't exchange another word; it is safe to assume that we are on the same page. Our only hope is that he gives up and leaves. What the actual fuck does he want? I wonder, as the ringing continues. How long had he been standing there, watching? What did he actually see? He probably couldn't distinguish our faces in the dark anyway.

I want to chase him away and pick up where we left off, but I'm ashamed that we got caught in the act. I wish I could be braver, but I can't stand the idea of being totally exposed in front of a potentially dangerous stranger.

Voilà! We both cower in the hallway waiting for a miracle to happen, unsure of what to do next. After about the tenth ring, the bell finally falls silent. I can hear Sébastien's sigh of relief as I snatch the curtains closed.

"I can't believe what just happened," says Sébastien, still shaken.

"This guy was insane," I reply, "or high on something strong." Noting the lack of vigor down under, I add, "It looks like this is the end for tonight." We go to our respective beds after a hug, the tension between us still palpable.

It turns out that dating your roommate is a risky matter (duh!). Shortly after our impromptu performance, Sébastien moved out, a necessary evil to regain a healthy balance in our relationship. I had made the mistake of pursuing too much passion too fast with a Brazilian guy I dated the previous year, and the memories of *that* drama were still fresh.

Even so, we soon realized that we were each at different life stages. I was Sébastien's first, whereas I had my first experience a long time ago. With time, we became and remain very close friends, despite the distance that separates us now, since my move to British Columbia five years ago.

Our friendship is not Sébastien's only legacy. I now avoid dating my roommates and make sure that my partners and I keep the curtains closed!

Lessons in Love-ology

SIMARBIR KAUR

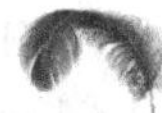

It's interesting how something as natural, and often accidental, as conceiving a child can suddenly feel like a full-blown, mission-critical science project when you're actually trying. How, when you start tracking your ovulation and menstrual cycles, and with only three days to conceive, even the forces of nature start acting up.

Before I get into the biology of how I conceived my child, I would like to explain how the chemistry of our lovemaking works. If I go through the chronicles of our intimate times in my mind, it has always been my husband's sudden urge that initiated the deed, drawing me in as well, making me crave intimacy during those terribly timed, impromptu arousals.

Time for some girl math. The probability of him

getting turned on is inversely proportional to the ease with which we can have sex. When getting intimate is the hardest, his desire will be the strongest. When we are comfortably lying in our bedroom, easily able to tango in the sheets, his hormones will flat-line while he binge-watches Netflix.

Some examples. When my husband and I went on a vacation with my mother-in- law, she insisted on keeping the door to our conjoined rooms open so she wouldn't feel alone. No sane couple would ever think of riding the horse of their sexual desires in such a situation. But we are different. When the lights went out, I whispered sweetly, "You looked smoking hot today in that yellow T-shirt. I wish we were alone tonight."

He gave me a quizzical look. "We are alone, babe. What do you mean?" Reading my face, he winked. "Oh, baby! Don't worry. She sleeps like a rock." He got so close to me that I could feel him getting turned on. Knowing my sweet spot, he started kissing my neck.

My desires were ignited, but I tried to be sensible. "Babe! The door is open," I said.

Undeterred, his kisses moved from my neck to my lips and his hands slowly started exploring the shape of my breasts. "We will be very quiet," he promised. His foreplay was punctuated with many more reassurances until I succumbed to desire. We both had the most wonderful time in bed that night, but the idea of my mother-in-law, waking up to our (definitely not quiet) moans and witnessing live porn starring her own son and daughter-in-law kept haunting me through all my orgasms.

On another occasion, we were on the topmost floor of the hotel where my friend was hosting her wedding reception. My I-know-all-the-isolated-corners of-a-hotel husband managed to secure a remote spot in a supposedly secluded hallway. The moonlight from the window at the end of the hallway illuminated the Sephora explosion on my face. "You look so beautiful, so gorgeous," he said, locking his eyes with me. "Let's do it, baby."

I pulled away and looked around in disbelief. "You have got to be kidding me. Here?"

"Yes, my love. It's perfect." He danced naughtily, making a sleazy gesture toward his crotch. "It's the perfect time to put my meat into your meat."

Little did he understand that, while his meat could be easily freed, my meat was very tightly wrapped inside a seventy-five fucking pound *lehenga*. NEWS FLASH: When you are dressed for an Indian wedding, getting to your vagina is like finding the missing piece of a jigsaw puzzle while blindfolded.

Failing to find any spot to kiss on my heavily bejewelled neck, he decided to revisit the curvature of my breasts and began pulling down the sleeve of my hand-embroidered blouse. Its velvety texture made it beautiful and shiny but tough to slide down. Fumbling to the other side, he encountered the battalion of safety pins used to set my *dupatta* (a long scarf). "How did they lock you inside that ensemble?" he giggled.

I laughed out loud, enjoying every second of playing hard to get. "It's not easy for you to get to your treasure," I said. I wanted to add that he was dealing with the result of six solid hours of hard work by the hair, makeup, and styling team. I was enjoying this lust vs *lehenga* game and wanted lust to win, so I started unfastening the back zip of my blouse. The clinking and clanking of my glass bangles and the jewelry dangling from every corner of my body made it tough. And noisy.

Defeated by the blouse, we decided to get down to business directly. He started to wrestle with the knot at my waist, which proved an adventure of its own. The silky string was tightly knotted to keep the heavy skirt from falling down, and we ended up tangling it even more. Laughter and desire both intensified.

If we couldn't get the lehenga down, we would lift it up. There were multiple layers, each of which seemed to be the last. "Peeling an onion is easier than this," my husband complained. "But we will get there, darling, don't worry."

After navigating gazillions of yards of fabric, my hard-working husband finally got his prize. "Eureka, I found it," he screamed when he felt the lace of my panties. The dark hallway that had echoed with our laughter was soon filled with moans.

We both claim that was the best sex we had ever had—so far. But one other incident deserves an honorable mention. I was cleaning the kitchen in a rush one morning when my husband stepped out of shower and wrapped his damp arms around my waist, his hands moving upward to my breasts. "I was thinking about you all the time in the shower," he breathed. I could feel things getting tighter between his legs as his kisses on my back became more urgent.

Lucky for him, he had used one of my favorite shower gels. Suddenly, the rush of the morning slowed down and my anxiety about getting to work on time disappeared. I could no longer hear the ticking of the clock. I turned around and whispered, "You smell so good, I want you more than you want me." A lacklustre morning became exciting.

I wish a woman's three-day ovulation periods were flexible enough to accommodate these unscripted, unplanned, unrehearsed and randomly timed sexual adventures. But no. Nature can't give us anything that easily. When we started the process of conceiving our child, I thought it would be easy, given our chemistry, sexual appetites, and our tendency to do it anytime, anywhere. But when I started scheduling everything around the results of my ovulation kits, science was suddenly thrown in the mix. We had to balance sexual chemistry with actual biology.

The pressure of my ovulation cycles adversely affected the spontaneity and frequency of our intimate acts. Math and biology got together to tarnish chemistry. The ovulation tracker app, Flo, suddenly became the anchor of our bedroom activities. Since making a baby takes teamwork, I gave my husband a complete rundown of how the app works. All our bedroom conversations suddenly centered around Flo and, over weeks of tracking cycles and checking cervical mucus, my husband's libido gradually evaporated. Even during those two-or-three day windows when the chance to conceive was high, he had lost interest. I'd become a couch covered in lace.

"Babe, do you want to have fun tonight?" I'd say, sliding down the strap of my lingerie.

"Your wish is my command," he would say, a child lured to a toy.

"The app says I am ovulating today," I whispered with a smile.

As if a switch had been flipped, he would slow down, kiss the back of my hand, and make an excuse. "Not one of my best nights, let's only cuddle tonight." I wish cuddling could make a baby.

There were countless nights like this, when Captain Flo would say "high chance of conceiving today" while the person who could make me pregnant watched continuous episodes of his favorite web series. I began to wonder if he was part of a secret binge-a-thon. Perhaps he was watching these back-to-back episodes to earn a reward, or to raise money for a good cause.

After weeks of his Netflix-induced showcoma, I decided to take action. When my ovulation stick told me I was ripe as a mango, I wrapped myself up like a present in my sexiest lingerie and replaced our cotton sheets and pillowcases with sleek, luxurious satin ones.

When my husband walked into our bedroom, his gaze shifted from the TV to me, posing on the bed. The silky lingerie and plunging lacy neckline earned me a standing ovation in his underpants. Slowly exploring the curves of my satin-clad body, he said, "Ooooh! This room is a mood. Did I accidentally check into our honeymoon suite?"

Making a conscious effort not to mention my

ovulation window, I made my voice husky. "Welcome to Lovers' Paradise. Tonight will be the best night of your life." Pulling him closer to me, I sensualized my voice even further. "Tonight, I want you truly, madly, and deeply inside me." What I wanted to say was, "Squeeze out the sperm, we need to make a baby tonight."

We learned a lot about fabrics that night. When I turned on my side, allowing my husband to kiss every inch of my back, I immediately, and repeatedly, slipped away from him, until I found myself clinging to the edge of the bed.

At first, I tried to ignore the problem. I centered myself again and closed my eyes, soaking in every second of passion, anticipating the next step. But now, with chemistry, biology, and even math working in our favour, physics entered the room for a lesson about friction. As my husband was sealing a kiss on the last few inches of my body, I slipped out from underneath him and onto our wooden floor.

I bruised my right hip, and nothing *fruitful* happened that night.

A month later, during which time not a single sexy look passed between us, it was time to try again. My hip had morphed from purple to blue, then finally green and yellow. But the father of my future children had lost all interest.

Instead, he'd discovered *Breaking Bad*, a gut-wrenching, emotionally intense drama series. I had to admit I was also hooked, and sitting down next to him in a pair of sweatpants, a bowl of popcorn between us, was much more appealing than trying to seduce any sperm out of him.

Still, I did not give up.

I continued to try. I bathed myself in every seductive scent that Bath & Body Works offered. I stripped to the point where neither Victoria nor I had any secrets left. When I finally succeeded in luring him away from his beloved screen to our bed (where our cotton sheets remained), I indulged him with a sensual massage before inviting him to do the same to my body. But no matter what we did, he failed to rise to the occasion. With a peck on my cheek and an apology, he went back to his show, caressing his new soulmate, the TV remote.

The only thing left to try was a seductive pole dance with knee-length silver boots. But when I ran that scenario in my mind, the pole always broke. Instead of a bruised hip, I foresaw breaking a bone. Try explaining that to an emergency room doctor.

After about six months, I decided it was time to throw biology, math, and physics out of the window to reignite the organic, intimate chemistry that would no longer be dictated by Captain Flo. I stopped talking about my cycles, deleted the Flo app from my phone and gave all the ovulation shenanigans a break. I just want to have a good time in bed again. Until, that is, I came up with a plan that, with the help of technology, made me feel like a sensual, female James Bond.

It was Friday night, and my husband had settled in bed watching a new series, *Vikings,* wearing a Bluetooth headset so I could read my book in peace. I was looking forward to an elevated, hybrid reading experience with both a printed copy and an audiobook of Mia Sheridan's *Archer's Voice*.

Now, you should know that *Archer's Voice* is a heartfelt romance between an introverted man and a woman haunted by past trauma who slowly heal each other. Its touching love story is punctuated with steamy lovemaking scenes. I read and listened, waiting for the moment when the book got to its sauciest passage.

As the protagonist, Bree, started to explain the amazing things that Archer was doing to her with his lips, my entire body heated up with desire for my man. When the narrator voice read ". . . he pressed his lips back to mine and brought his hands up," I paused the audio, selected my husband's headset from the list of Bluetooth devices on my phone, pressed play, and watched as the audio seeped into his ears. As I waited, I deleted my AirPods' device name from my phone.

My heart pounding, I paused his show. "My AirPods got disconnected from my phone," I said in my best I-don't-know-what's-happening voice.

"Yes, because my headset got connected to your phone," he replied. I stifled a giggle.

My husband is good with technology and enjoys fixing things for me. As he started troubleshooting, his hands busy reconnecting my earpieces to my phone, he had no choice but to listen to the audiobook. To my delight, he started focusing on the audio much more intently. I overheard the narrator's voice continuing, ". . . It felt so good that I moaned again, pressing my hips upward into his hard body. I could feel his erection hard and thick, and I wiggled until it was pressed right where I needed it, the heat of it radiating through his jeans and the thin fabric of my linen shorts."

My husband's interest in fixing the technical problem disintegrated. Soon, he was no longer holding my phone or the AirPods. I waited a little longer, watching him respond to his own arousal.

"Oh, I see you're listening to my book," I said with feigned nonchalance. From the corner of my eye, I could see him turn toward me, shifting the sheets and looking at me with the lustful gaze I longed for. My heart started racing, but I wanted to appear innocent and ignorant.

His mood shifted 180 degrees as he reached for the TV remote and switched off his show. I could see in his eyes that I was now his feature film.

My need for him was pulsing furiously into desperation. I closed the final distance between us and felt his body tremble with passion.

"You're so beautiful," he whispered, pulling me into a deep embrace while curling his fingers through my hair.

I gazed directly into his eyes. "I feel beautiful when you look at me."

His kiss was passionate, and we were finally rising high on this riptide of sexual energy suppressed for months. His soft, trembling fingers traced every curve of my body, finding new sensual spots neither of us knew existed. And with every whispering breath, he looked deep into my eyes as though he might lose himself inside of me.

When the audiobook narrator concluded the chapter, "And nothing had ever felt more right," we both smiled as we removed our headphones. Just like Bree and Archer, we had found each other. Relief at reinstating our romance and realizing how much we had longed for each other filled my heart with joy.

Not only was our chemistry back, but biology finally joined in with math and physics. Five weeks after that incredible night, that night that was about the two of us and nothing else, two pink lines confirmed that we had succeeded in our mission of conceiving a baby!

Boyfriend Duties

DEAN SLUGGER JONES

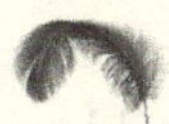

She texts me and tells me she misses me and my color-changing clit.

She texts me and tells me she wants to choke on it while my cum drips down her chin.

She texts me and tells me she wants me to cum inside of her.

I like to imagine my cum inside of her. I think about it all the time. While driving, walking, writing, eating, laughing, sweating, flowing, playing, cleaning, I'm scheming ways to make her drip. Ways to get my dick wet. Envisioning her mouth covered in my cum. My mouth covered in hers. I mix my spit around my mouth like I would her cum. I think about her collecting shower water in her mouth, spitting it into mine, and letting it drip down and out of my mouth while she watches less than an inch from my face, her fingers spreading me. I think about her fingers.

She has strong hands. Virgo hands. I noticed them the night our lives collided. I sat behind her and her lover at the queer bar and watched her knead into her lover's shoulders while she licked their ear and whispered to them. *Stop being so curious. So turned on. You shouldn't want her. She's probably not even polyamorous like us. Stop watching her fucking hands.* I scolded myself and held my convictions until she pushed her front body onto my back and her pelvis onto my ass as we walked out the door. A two-person conga line. Her hand wrapped round me, gripping my outer hip.

Fuuuuuck. Her hands. Her hands! I bit my tongue, grateful she couldn't see my blush or feel my wet, hot panic.

Months later, she texts me a selfie of her in a shark hat. It covers all but her eyes and mouth. I'm at work playing cars with a three-year-old when I see it. She looks ridiculous and sexy, and in a matter of seconds, I'm wet and twitching. *Great, I'm hard at work. I am no better than a teenage boy.* Despite my clit-dick standing at less than two inches, I fidget and put a pillow over my lap. Put my phone away, chug water, and keep playing. A foolish attempt to cool this pulsing clit of mine so desperately seeking her mouth. This clit of mine so desperate.

When you go on testosterone, everything changes. How you express emotions. The sound of your voice. The way your moods swing. How hair grows, where your hair grows, its texture. The shape of your jaw and hips. Your feet, hands, shoulders, and ribs broaden. Your muscles shift and harden. One morning you wake up feeling like Buffy's little brother who beefed up practically overnight, suddenly equipped to kill. Your clit gradually grows into a little dick. Its lid becomes foreskin. The walls of your vaginal canal thicken and harden. Your labia plumps up and gets hard like balls when you're turned on. Your hard little dick, or clit, twitches and pulses like a penis that's been freed and is begging to be touched. Instantaneously, you're an uncut king, so horny all the time it's as if you're continuously ovulating.

It can be exhilarating to be so aroused. Uncomfortable and weird, too. Uncharted territory for a person who spent most of their life as a cautious demisexual cycling with the moon. Meaning, I only wanted to fuck someone when my heart pounded for them just as hard as my pussy. Without that, sex was hardly on my mind, even when fertile. The opening of my heart was the key to releasing my chastity. On testosterone, my desire to fuck is constant, but my desire to be promiscuous remains minimal. I still prefer a heart-pounding dick throb over a casual fuck.

Three months on testosterone and into our courtship, she fucked me for the first time. I hadn't been able to make myself come for weeks. Instead, I'd writhe into a frustrated ball of overstimulation. It was almost painful, how badly I needed a release I couldn't access. Like blue balls or something. Multiple times a day, I tried and failed. With all this new surface area to explore, I didn't know what part of my cunt to breathe into. I didn't know how hard or fast or tender a touch my clit needed.

I used to suction my dildo onto stacked yoga blocks and ride it while pressing my vibrator on my clit until I passed out; now, I couldn't even handle my own fingers inside of me, let alone my vibrator. Horny as a teenager and no way to release. But when she fucked me? I came with ease. Multiple fingers and multiple orgasms later, I bled all over her white bed. White sheets. White pillowcases. White blankets. White walls. White rug. I hadn't bled in months because of testosterone, and, despite dysphoria from bleeding, seeing her hands cum-covered and mixed with my blood turned me on all over again. I wanted to kiss it. Lick it off. Ravenous.

BOYFRIEND DUTIES

The first time I made myself come with her in mind, I was driving my car away from the parking lot of the restaurant with the couch in front of the fireplace. The couch where I learned just how far I'll toe the line between public displays of affection and exhibitionism. Where I would have fucked her if the room had been darker. If she was ready for it. Where she pulled my hands off her ass, slid her tongue out from the back of my mouth, and whispered, "I don't understand all these feelings I have for you. It's like I'm a teenager again or something, not a forty-year-old woman."

"Is that a bad thing?" I asked, always nervous that our ten-year age gap would become a problem.

"I don't know," she said, placing her hands on her body like she was searching for herself before sliding back onto the couch and into my arms.

I hid my face in her neck and laughed, confessing into her hair. "I feel like a teenager with you, too. Second puberty has me all dick and no brains."

She sighed and kissed me until the host came and put new logs on the fire. "It's not a bed, ladies," he joked. I was so engrossed that I didn't realize he had misgendered me until days later.

That was the night I learned just how hard a growing clit will buzz, just how loud it will beg. The night I finally started to understand how a grown-ass man can get caught up in the messes his dick makes and the things it demands.

Grinding on her thigh and grabbing her tits. *Buzz*.

Biting her bottom lip and pressing her up against her truck. *Buzz*.

Waddling back to my car with soaked boxers and wet pants and a clit so hard my entire body was a' *buzz buzz buzzing* so hard I . . .

The first time I cried in front of her, we were in a dark room at the Ace Hotel after an evening of karaoke. While two double-sided dildos sat untouched in her bag, I cried and cried because *of course* God had to make me a neurodivergent queer trans boy who can mask his sensitivities until they build to such an intensity I combust and am left inconsolable, unresponsive, and unrecognizable in my overstimulation. I shut down. I can't hear you. I get irritable and mean. I pull my knees into my chest and squeeze into the tiniest ball possible, rocking on my tailbone. I ugly cry. In short, I throw a tantrum. To me, it feels like becoming a monster. A werewolf on a full moon or something.

I'm not violent when this happens, but I do get sharp. Sharp with words. Sharp with glances. Sharp with my movements. It doesn't happen nearly as often as it did before I started to transition, which is when my body started to feel like it was mine. And I always try to wait until I am home alone before I burst. A precaution I developed out of fear of being abandoned as a guy who suddenly needs so much support. A fear of causing harm.

That night at the Ace Hotel, with its ambient decibel level between 70 and 85, my threshold for stimulation decreased as my need to escape and my inability to express it increased. It was all the noise on the streets mixed with all the people in and out of the karaoke bar and the roar of conversations held in-between and during songs. All the alcohol. The lack of weed. The pressure I put on myself for her friends to like me. To not be too much, this new guy in her life.

I require myself to be charming, and generous, and handsome. I stand closest to the road when we walk on the sidewalk. Hold her bag. Hold her drink. Hold her hand. Kiss her face. Take the pictures. I need to prove I know how to function like a *normal* person. Prove I am the kind of guy they know she deserves. That I know she deserves. I never told her that I get like this. Overstimulated and inconsolable. I never know how or when to bring it up with people, and, before I could warn her, before I could tell her what I might need, before she could run, there she was holding me at 1:00 am while tears and boogers gathered on my face and her T-shirt.

With a shaky voice and body, I tried to explain. "This happens to me sometimes. It all becomes too much. The noise. The conversations. The vibrations in my body. My hyper-vigilance and my mean inner critic. I hope I didn't ruin your night. I hope they liked me. I hope you had fun. I'm sorry if this is too much. If I'm too much. I'm sorry we're not playing with the toys you brought . . ."

I kept crying because I had to release somehow. Because all I wanted to do was come with her, clit to clit. Legs wrapped. Double-sided dildo snatched up in us. Buzzing. Instead, I was surrendering. Showing her what I always keep hidden.

"You have nothing to apologize for," she reassured me. "You did great, baby. You're doing great. They all loved you. And I love you. Cry as much as you need."

In the morning, when I fuck her, I know without a doubt that everyone on the eighth floor of the Ace Hotel knows my name.

She texts me and tells me she needs to feel me cum so she can sleep well.

She texts me and tells me she needs me to fill her mouth and pussy at once.

She texts me and tells me she wants her mouth to fill with salivation for my salty fingers and sweet treats.

Before I met her, I spent a year celibate. Before that, four years having sex almost exclusively with cis men. Before that, very boring, vanilla sex with my sweet, genderqueer, masculine-presenting, Pisces ex-fiancé, who was very comfortable with only touching me, which was all I could tolerate back then. I don't know if it was their true preference to be a touch-me-not, their own body dysphoria. Or their respect for the unresolved childhood sexual trauma that I refused to discuss. But touching dicks and pussies (even my own) was difficult to do. It doesn't really matter. What matters was that my fiancé was on their knees to please me and make me feel safe. Much as I am, now, with her. The first time I made her come, she cried, as she often does. And I held her, as I always do.

Before I met her, I'd never searched "blow job" on a porn website. Shit, I'd never typed *anything* into a porn website. But:

There is a bench in her shower facing the shower head. A month after our first fuck, and about four months on T, she pushed me down onto the bench and knelt over my lap. While her mouth held, sucked, licked, pulled, and devoured me, I watched hot water cascade down her spine between her ass cheeks. I watched her mouth suck me and noticed that, for the first time, my hard clit was big enough to stick out between my lips. I lifted my hips and spread myself further. Enchanted by my firmness. My ability to penetrate her. "I can feel you pulsing and twitching in my mouth. You keep getting harder," she moaned.

Her teeth tickling my tip. I held her head down and imagined myself growing large enough to tap her tonsils. An animalistic need to be sucked and licked ferociously like I'm Lil Wayne or something. I fucked her face and slid myself to the edge of the bench to welcome her fingers inside of me. I fucked her face and begged her to fuck me harder. Letting my puberty-stricken vocal chords break in their moaning without thought of embarrassment. Each time she hit my G-spot I moaned in crackles.

Every time she fucks me, I come differently. Different from the last time and different from how I used to. Before my clit got so big, before my prostate grew into my pussy, hardening me from the inside out.

I used to desire being the lover who was pulled and yanked and stretched and bent in all kinds of directions. Who was left whimpering in painful delight. Who released control and thought and gave their body over to another for however long I could last. However long they could handle me. I used to only want gentle touches on my tiny clit. I'd come from such a feathered touch I feared boring my lovers despite how much I'd twitch for them. Sometimes I feared their boredom so much, I'd fake enjoyment in their hard-tongued licks and too-firm fingertips and ignore my need for tenderness. I'd lie in bed with my lovers with the intention of giving like a sex doll. Sprawled out however they desired. Face down, ass up, receiving. Always receiving like a good girl does.

Porn made me nauseous. Watching anyone fuck who I didn't have feelings or desire for made me gag. Now I watch men with girthy dicks fuck all kinds of people's mouths all rough while I fuck myself and imagine I am fucking her with my dick like that. Grabbing her like that. Bending her over and teasing her with my tip like that. Slapping her ass like that. Talking her through it like that. Edging her on like that. Coming with her like that. And I do fuck her like that. With my fingers and hands and mouth and toys until we're giggling in relief and covered in each other's sweat and come, eating ice cream or popsicles or cookies in bed.

The first time she told me she loved me, she was drunk and I was stoned. We were in bed at her friend's house in Brooklyn, a basement they all referred to as the sex dungeon. She kept saying, "Do you know?" Based on her blush, her eye contact, and the energy of the room, I did know. In fact, I had known for weeks. Each time we made eye contact while fucking, one of us was trying not to blurt it out. Usually, the one closer to climax. That night, I made her tell me between fits of giggles.

I wanted her to be the first one to say it because she was the one who resisted being with me when we first met. We spent months talking poetics via texts. Spent months dancing around the idea of acting on our desires. Months of her not being sure, and me being very sure and happy to follow her lead. I had no desire to ignore my wish to hold her and learn her heart tender-like. By the time she asked me if I wanted to go out, I felt I could collapse in relief.

The closest I came to confession was a week or so before she let it slip. When she had my head pushed up into her headboard in her cathedral. I call her house her cathedral because of the tall ceilings. The way the rooms echo. The way moonlight trickles in. How frequently I'm on my knees in surrender. To her. To us. To pleasure. Moonlight poured onto us while she fucked me slow. My legs up and wide, one over her shoulder, the other behind my head. Her mouth teased my dick. Her fingers filled me. She had me so outside myself and inside my cunt all I could do was whisper, "Baby."

In the sex dungeon, after her schoolgirl-like, giggling-fit confession, I kissed the rouge of her blushing cheeks. Nuzzled into her neck. Pulled her ass deeper into my pelvis. Rested my lips on her ear, held her still, whispered, "I've been in love with you since you first snored and drooled on my chest in your cathedral. It was a full moon, and my arm was asleep, and I kissed your forehead and I prayed out loud, Please, let this love last."

We rolled over and lay there, perfect spoons, my left thigh creeping between her legs, her bottom lip between my teeth. I felt her heartbeat under my palms. Smelled her heat, felt her damp cunt through her sleep shorts. Despite her being fully clothed, I thrust and thrust and thrust my thigh between her legs while she ground her pussy up and down and round. With one arm around her throat, forcing her to look at me, my other hand gripped and pulled her thigh, slapped her ass. I held her gaze and spoke sweetly to her, "That's it, baby. Fuck me just like that. Breathe, baby. There you go. That's it. Get what you need, baby. Give me your come, baby. Yes. That's it. Good job, baby. I've got you." Come-covered and whimpering, she fell asleep in my arms, her drool on my chest.

Two days later, she texted me: I think I have a yeast infection.

I immediately felt guilty for fucking her so hard with her sleep shorts on: I'm sorry, baby. I should've taken your shorts off the other night. Made you pee before you passed out.

My phone pinged instantly: Never apologize for fucking me.

I brought itch cream and over-the-counter pussy treatments to her at work. I walked into her shop smiling, the products balanced haphazardly in my hands. I let them fall on the counter, pressed my palms, and lifted myself up to kiss her. "Remember, don't insert the egg into your pussy till bedtime. Let me know if you want help," I teased. I kissed her one more time and raced out the door, late for work, without a care.

I drove away guilty with joy, laughing as I texted her: I feel like a real boyfriend, buying you yeast infection medicine after fucking you too hard.

Ending Lockdown

ANASTASIA SOROKA, LPC

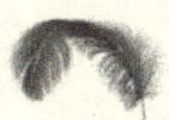

How do you know you can trust your partner with the vulnerable parts of you? The pieces of you that you're afraid to admit exist?

I was a sex educator through college and am now a therapist who specializes in couples' and intimacy work within trauma, and I'm only beginning to figure out the answers to these questions myself.

It's been a wild, uncomfortable ride.

When I was in graduate school, I met a cute, smooth-talking engineer with double the confidence of all my previous partners. We spent a total of five years together, the last two during the Covid-19 lockdown. Lockdown was our downfall, but my salvation. He said all the right things and talked about the importance of safety in relationships. I remember my heart racing and my anxiety tumbling around in my chest. Finally, my chance to tell the truth. My truth. He can hear me; I can be safe, I thought. The joke was on me. He missed it all. It was like I offered him a slice of banana cream pie while all he cared about was stuffing his own banana. I ended up with cream all over my face.

I'm getting ahead of myself, though, so let me explain. I am self-diagnosed with vaginismus, which is when the vaginal canal tightens up whenever anything is inserted into it. Imagine a waterslide. Everyone is having a blast. But when it's your turn, the water pressure drops, the tunnel shrinks, and you get friction burn all the way down. By the time you drop into the pool, everyone is screaming in excitement, and you're begging for it to be over.

I spent my life avoiding anything going up there, including feminine hygiene products. I quit the swim team when puberty hit because I literally could not use a tampon and was too embarrassed to tell anyone. I assumed this was a normal part of who I was. I was a badass in other areas of my life, and there was nothing to be done about it, so I did my best to ignore it.

When I started dating Smooth-Talking Engineer, however, he took the mentality that my vaginismus was a problem that needed to be solved. That *I* was a problem that needed to be solved.

Over the first few years we were together, he'd offer solutions: "Maybe you should go try another doctor?" Or "Let's figure this out so we can continue to have fun." (Read: so he could continue to have fun). The message was clear—I was broken, and it was my job to figure it out.

I worked hard to make him happy. I went to four different doctors and each gave me the same four solutions:

"It's a yeast infection." (It was never a yeast infection.)

"Here's some medication." (Tried it. Didn't help.)

"Use more lube." (I assure you, I used handfuls, buckets, waterfalls of lube!)

"Birth control must be wrong; let's change it again." (NO!)

During lockdown, I began working on my couples specialization. I learned how to be curious, how to fight fairly, and how to grow and heal together as a couple.

I would burst out of my office like a scientist who discovered the cure for cancer and desperately show my partner the research. "Look! This can help us! Let's work on us!"

He, on the other hand, would stare at me, deadpan, instantly defensive, and would even try to blame the research. "Every time you learn something new, you point out something else wrong with us. Who are you going to listen to? These people with decades of experience, or me?"

How did I not see that red flag? I should have run. I didn't.

Looking back, maybe I should have believed him, this engineer with no mental health knowledge or interest in having deep conversations. Or foreplay. Maybe he was onto something. Maybe my problem was that I kept learning new things, and if I could have stopped thinking for myself, we would have had a happy and healthy relationship. Unfortunately for us, I'm just too damn smart, and I refused to make myself smaller for anyone. Instead, I put off intimacy as much as possible.

And then, during the pandemic, intimacy became easier to stave off because we were in lockdown with four other roommates. We did family dinners instead of date nights. And I was never alone, which used to be my nightmare, but soon became my armor, saving me from the pain. Occasionally, my partner would take motorcycle rides through the mountains with his buddies (his soulmates) while I relaxed at home with my dogs (my soulmates). Once home, he would strip naked the second our bedroom door was closed and helicopter his dick around, making me laugh. But then the pressure would start.

Over time, he became impatient for sex. And the more impatient he became, the more I enjoyed spending time with our roommates. Saying, "Let's play a board game" instead of going to bed early. Pushing him away with "No, no, really, it doesn't bother me that you want to play your video game together all night, have a great time!" Just so I could have some peace. I really should have paid attention to that red flag, too, but I was surviving lockdown the best I could and making friends along the way.

One day, frustrated, I asked, "Why aren't you doing more to make me feel safe? Why don't you care about connection? Why don't you want to spend time with me?"

Without even a second to process, Smooth-Talking Engineer confidently stated, "I'm not the one with the problem. I'm doing everything right. If there's a problem, it's on your side, so you are the one who needs to change."

These words triggered my strong, independent self and she promptly bitch-slapped me into reality. It was the wake-up call I needed.

My partner was right. I was the one who needed to change. And I did, by leaving him behind. I'm a great therapist, and I suddenly realized I was helping everyone but myself.

I felt like a woman in a chick flick who finally

realizes she doesn't need a man to be happy. The universe cued up the inspirational background music as I chose myself and walked away.

Something you should know about me is that I'm biromantic, but demisexual. Which means, if you want to get in my pants and want me to want you there, you have to make an effort to navigate conflict. Sounds obvious, but Smooth-Talking Engineer never got the hint. I am the expert in my own life, and while I'm not a medical doctor, I sure as hell knew a lot more about sexuality than the doctors I was meeting with.

I started to explore diagnoses and finally found the answer that fit: vaginismus. The thing about vaginismus is that it can be treated and healed, but a fear of being out of control can make it worse. Imagine trying to get a massage with a sunburn. The massage therapist knows exactly what they're doing and thinks it will feel good for you, but all it does is sting, hurt, and make you tense up.

I am also a recovering perfectionist with strong control issues, so when I figured things out, I was not surprised this is how my body manifested its anxiety.

I talked to my newest doctor about it and was finally given insight into all the ignorance I was met with previously. "We are only taught three solutions in medical school. If it's not one of those three, I can't help you."

With that, it all made sense. They couldn't diagnose me because they weren't taught how to, even if I was giving them the answer! Relief hit me like that bucket of lube was always supposed to.

I wasn't crazy.

I moved forward, found my voice again, and promised myself I would never let another person hurt me for the sake of their fun.

Free from the lockdown and the relationship, I began running daily, climbing weekly, and intentionally choosing myself. I told a friend, "I don't need a relationship, but if the universe sends me someone, I'll be open to exploring it."

That's when I met him. A beautiful, blue-eyed man with matching blue hair in the bouldering cave at the gym where we problem-solved an orange V5 together. Laughed a little. But I wanted to be single, so I decided to leave it at that first meeting and not explore more.

He, however, refused to let go that easily.

I remember packing up my bag and feeling his piercing gaze on my back. I pretended not to watch him as he stood up and joined me once again. I could feel the universe challenging my agreement to be open. He asked for my contact information, and I agreed. I figured he would, at least, be a fun climbing buddy for the summer. Later, he told me, "Your intelligence drew me in; I had to know more about you."

We texted for three days straight, talking about everything from travel to blacksmithing. We made a plan to climb with friends the following week, and he asked to see me—alone—before we climbed.

I remember being curious, but ambivalent. *Why not?*

We met in a park, with the plan to walk and talk until it was time to climb. He showed up in a brightly colored button-down and donut socks. He was carefree, authentic, and comfortable in his body. Now I was the one who wanted to know more.

To pay his way through college, this 100% straight man was a go-go dancer at a gay bar. "Everyone goes straight for the butt," he laughed. "But it let me dance, and it was good money."

This beautiful and wholesome go-go dancer paused at a picnic table. "Do you want to dance?"

I nodded in excitement. *I always wanted a dance partner.*

He played the song "Kiss Me" by Lola Jane. A slow, romantic, Latin song. We danced, our bodies moving together, our souls connecting. And it was so chick-flick cheesy that I wanted to throw up.

Being with him felt so easy that I rolled my eyes at

the universe. *Seriously? I wasn't expecting someone so quickly.* I could feel the universe laughing at me, like a girlfriend who'd set me up.

Our first month together felt much like that first dance: easy-going, low pressure, with us being pulled towards each other.

By then, I'd had the two pandemic years to convince myself that emotional intimacy was the answer, and that it's a part of my identity. I would not settle for someone who makes it all about them. I needed to test the waters. I drafted a text, opening up about the pressure, the pain, and my low sex drive (especially when there are life stressors). I shared my need to slow down and take pressure off. I meant it when I said I wouldn't spend the rest of my life in pain for someone else, and if he wasn't willing to go slow with me, he should find someone else.

The vulnerability in my text terrified me. I left it as a draft all day. I panic-texted my friend, "Am I really doing this? Is it too early? What if he can't accept me?"

My friend reminded me, "If he doesn't accept you, you don't want him anyway. You wanted to be single."

Oh yeah.

I hit send. I panicked some more. I made a plan to flee the country and start fresh, somewhere new. I've always loved Italy, but it would be hard to transport a dog across the ocean. How about Canada? I could drive my belongings north, get my PhD, and become an asexual recluse.

A few minutes later, Go-Go Dancer replied, "Of course, I will explore at whatever speed you want or need, just tell me where you'd like to start." I burst into tears. I cried from the flood of safety I felt and for every past version of myself that felt pressured or rushed or broken. He saw me and accepted me.

What the fuck, Universe?

It has been over three years now since that text exchange, and I can tell you that Go-Go Dancer meant it. We've explored together, slowed down together, and I found that sometimes I want to speed up. I finally learned why people say sex is fun. I don't have pain anymore, and in the moments where my mind wanted sex but my body wasn't ready, we stopped immediately.

I still cry sometimes, but not from pain. More often than not, we laugh. Together. We laugh because my present is finally allowing me to heal in a way I never thought possible from my past. It's almost ridiculous, but the tears are coming out of me as I type. But it's okay, I can laugh at the tears, too.

There is no pressure, no expectation. I am never

made to feel guilty or broken for not being on his schedule. Whenever the pressure resurfaces, I tell my Go-Go Dancer what the voice is saying, which is, "You haven't had sex in a while, he is going to leave you."

And every time, without fail, he replies, "There's no rush," and does a body roll for emphasis.

If we've been too busy or haven't been able to connect, he reassures me, "Of course you're not in the mood, we haven't been able to spend time together emotionally. I don't want you to be anything but yourself." My pain is gone, and I have never felt safer.

Together, we stopped caring about the outcomes, or how often we physically engage in sex, because the intimacy and safety make everything we do together so much fun. We dance in the kitchen, make out on the couch, and make sure to touch each other's butts as often as physically possible—I hope to one day outnumber the random hands who have touched his perfectly round cheeks from his gay-bar days.

I needed to trust myself, and to trust my body when it was telling me no. Now that I can do that, I can finally hear my body saying, "Yes." This is a freedom we can both enjoy.

If there comes a time when I'm in the mood and he isn't, he can kiss me and say, "I'm too hot, not tonight."

I'll reply with, "How dare you? Don't you understand how rare it is that I'm horny?" We will laugh and move on together, as a team, finding an activity that works for both of us. Before my go-go dancer, I didn't know this kind of safety existed. I didn't know this kind of connection was an option. And I certainly didn't know a butt like his existed.

Now, I never want to go back.

Wouldn't you want the same?

Panty Vending Machine

SOPHIA MCGOVERN

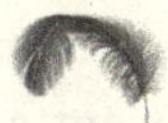

I'm sitting in Amsterdam, waiting for my tiny fried dim sum at an Asian tapas restaurant. Beautiful people on bikes (so many bikes!) glide past the window on cobblestones, so different from the melting asphalt of Phoenix, Arizona. I flew here for some solo writing time in one of the world's most incredible cities. And having planned this trip for months, no guy was going to get in the way.

My shiny new relationship had begun when a pack of male artists in their thirties crowded around me and my friend at a poetry reading in downtown Phoenix. A year out of college, we'd hoped to be feature poets someday. And we loved to flirt.

At the time, I was in my seventh year of on-and-off-again with my First Everything boyfriend. But here was

Jeff, a journalist. A journalist with a girlfriend, who chatted about the kinds of books that made you want to pick up a pen.

A few months later, while First Everything was busy snorting away the stress of his doctoral program, Jeff's girlfriend dumped him. He was farm-sitting nearby for a metal-working artist he'd once written about, who had horses and an iguana that was older than me. Did I want to stop by with some of my writing?

Although it was innocent at first, talking all night and reading each other's work turned out to be more intimate than any hookup. I could feel how much he cared about me, but something told me we'd either drown together or build something that could last. Both were frightening.

While First Everything was still too messed up to take my calls, Jeff threw a party at the farm. All the coolest creative folk gathered under the stars, between the horse stables and the goat pen. It was going smoothly until the clock struck midnight, a horse bit our dancer friend, and my poetry mother's nonverbal son mangled all the owner's beaded jewelry while stimming.

After everyone left, I helped Jeff clean up the heaping mess. And then, I let it happen: sex in the way I asked for, with no kissing or eye contact. On a filthy rug that wasn't mine. Or even, really, his. The next day, the owner of the farm kicked us out, and I broke up with First Everything. Jeff and I kept seeing each other and, at some point that neither of us can remember, we became official.

I soon found myself at my own apartment, packing for Amsterdam and bawling my eyes out like a teenager reading *The Fault in Our Stars* for the first time. Did that mean I was falling for this ridiculous red-headed man, ten years older than me and filled with wild stories? Many of them about other women?

Jeff did all he could to dry my tears. "I got something for you," he said with a flourish as he held out a pair of panties at eye level, beaming. "Straight from my couch cushions! Now you can remember all our good times while you're away." He wriggled his eyebrows, but I could only glare. The striped Victoria's Secret hipsters were not mine.

Sure, in a club, I would wear next to nothing and melt into anonymity in a steamy mass of dancers. But under the pitiless fluorescent lighting of a Victoria's Secret, the peppy advertising and multitude of choices unfailingly sent me into a panic; I'd never left that place with so much as a bra.

I knew Jeff hadn't cheated on me. He just wasn't the type to clean under couch cushions. Which is why I could see the faintest trace of white-cheddar-cheese-puff dust on the trim of the undies. No. The panties belonged to Jeff's ex-girlfriend, who is nice, wonderful, smaller, and much more well-known in the art community than I was.

Obviously, I hate her.

"It's fine. You thought they were mine," I said. But even when I landed in Amsterdam and settled myself into this entirely other continent, I couldn't help but wonder what other good times that couch still remembered.

To calm myself, I lit a joint and, moments later, imagined myself pulling pair after pair of other women's bright, overpriced panties out of the mustard-yellow, ratty velvet cushions of Jeff's mangy couch.

In my mind, I first clawed a lacy pink bikini, belonging to the blond actress whose voice sounded like a Kia car alarm. Then an olive-green boy short for the hip bike girl who liked to be on top. Then a silky black thong from the musician who conjured her next bass line from reverse cowgirl.

I gagged at the high-waisted, organic-cotton pair from the earth mama who gives the best head, based on astrological signs.

While I blew smoke out the window of my tiny Dutch hotel room, Jeff called, waxing poetic about his love spanning any ocean. I said nothing as my thoughts circled the imaginary heap of orphaned panties at my feet.

Finally, he asked, "Don't you remember the other night?"

We'd had sex in his grungy apartment, and I let myself go, relaxing into him. When he thought I was asleep, he whispered, "I love you," into my bedhead. I guffawed like a lady, and he covered his face with his hands. This man felt all his feelings out loud, and by God, there were a lot of them—all meant for me and all wonderful. Instead of going home that night, and instead of returning those words, I slept in his arms.

But that was before his couch puked up his ex's unmentionables.

"Have you found any more treasures in that disgusting couch of yours?"

"So, I've cleaned my whole apartment, and no." When I didn't congratulate him for his lack of lingerie, he continued. "I meant what I said the other night. I don't know if I should say this yet, but you're amazing, and I want to spend the rest of my life with you."

With that, my hotel room filled with a weed-tinged warm glow. Maybe this thing between us could happen. Maybe a future was waiting for us, one where we could weather the chaos and thrive.

That was a week ago, and now, at the end of my

time in Amsterdam, when the server sets down my dim sum and another Brand Weizen, I sip the fruity beer and smile.

Even though it's my last night in this incredible place, I'm excited to return to the staggering desert heat. Because when my plane lands, Jeff will be waiting for me. We'll write and travel the world together. First, though, when I step into his arms, I'll tell him those three big little words.

But fuck that couch.

Rare White Buffalo

WENDY L. SCHMIDT

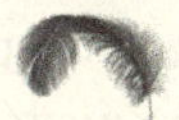

When it came to sex, conversations with my husband often circled the same two issues.

He said: I want it twice a week with *à la carte* offerings.

She said: I'll counter your offer with once every two weeks, with specialty items bestowed only on birthdays, anniversaries, and secular holidays.

After being married for twenty-five years, I thought we'd passed through all the itchy phases. But, as soon as I saw the vintage red ragtop roll into the driveway, I knew something was up. A catty neighbor spotted it too and couldn't wait to hiss the dreaded words: *midlife crisis*.

My marriage was living on borrowed time. The

ending began with his Mustang-mistress and finally concluded with a mundane household chore.

I was placing clean boxer shorts into my husband's top drawer when I happened upon a brown paper bag. Curiosity and a nagging sense of suspicion got the better of me. I knew nothing good could ever come from a brown paper bag hidden in the back of an underwear drawer. My fingers faltered as I dared to invade my husband's private space. *Serves him right*, I told myself, *for expecting me to fold his underwear*.

A quick rip of the lone staple holding the bag closed, and out spilled the sordid contents. Books, but not just any books. How-to sex manuals: *How to Please Your Partner, Hot Sex, Down and Dirty, The Guide to Getting Some.*

Clearly, none of these were meant for me. So who was the intended target?

I didn't need Miss Marple to help me solve the mystery. A few clicks of the keyboard and I found more clues in the form of personal emails. Friendly at first, the letters quickly progressed to provocative.

After reading the last of their correspondence, I stared at the screen for a full fifteen minutes, until I felt sick to my stomach. Not only was my husband having an affair, his partner turned out to be the wife of his best friend from college. They lived in different states, but that hadn't stopped them. Confused, fearful, and angry, especially at the double betrayal, I felt something else too: the need to confront this one head on.

That evening, I watched and listened as my husband attempted to tap-dance his way through the three stages of scoundrelism: denial, righteous indignation, and fear of exposure. Finally, he owned up to the emails then, because I wanted to know just how far things had gone, he added the details of their phone sex and regressed adolescent fantasies. No regret, no willingness to take the blame. Only the cold reality that this hidden part of my partner was completely unknown to me. He could have shared the sex manuals with me, but instead sought to share them with someone outside our marriage.

I wondered how many more secrets I would find if I scratched the surface.

I was a middle-aged woman coming off a long-term relationship, unused to being on my own. And while the big decisions were daunting, the little ones were heartbreaking. Staring into the abyss of singlehood, I asked myself: should I pursue a second chance at love and marriage? Or was I doomed to repeat the same mistakes?

I felt like a wilted wallflower, blindly walking through a dense field of dating apps. Even with my limited experience, I could tell that the profiles were too good to be true. After swiping left on hundreds, if not thousands, of men holding fish, men with cheap hair plugs, and men claiming to have practiced every position in the *Kama Sutra,* I came to the informed conclusion that coupling wasn't what I wanted at all.

What came next was eye-opening. Many of my married friends began to cancel the unconventional older woman, and odd girl out, that I had suddenly become.

FRIEND: Oh dear, I didn't know you were planning on coming to the dinner on your own. We want even numbers, you understand.

ME: Is this an actual un-vitation?

FRIEND: I think the book club is a better fit for you. We're reading *Big Little Lies* this month.

This was not an isolated incident. Despite all the rejection, I felt the growing need to be my authentic self. And I instinctively knew this wasn't going to happen for me with a man stuck to my side. I was beginning to see that true love was mostly a fantasy. And if it did exist, it must be like spotting a rare white buffalo. A miracle. A fairytale. Or a gift that only a few blessed couples are chosen to receive, while others are left searching every randy app or random encounter for their perfect mate.

I was no longer the naive young woman I was when

I was first married. What I wanted, what I needed, was perhaps a friend-with-benefits, no strings or rings attached. I soon discovered there were vanishingly few examples of this kind of partnership among aging baby boomers. Even when the men I met started off enthusiastic at my proposal of unattached sex, they all soon wanted more. Someone—me—to take over their domestic needs. As though sex and vacuuming were somehow inextricable.

Some of the men I met wanted a wife. All wanted a mother. And while a few did want a friend-with-benefits, unfortunately the benefits were more along the lines of meal preparation, picking up socks, and washing and folding—you guessed it—his underwear. I wasn't about to go down that clothesline again.

It was shocking to realize, even after the 70s women's lib movement, that the ideal of woman as wife/mother/whore was still alive and kicking. Men from my generation still wanted all three in one woman.

Oh, sure, they talked the talk. But their support grew out of shallow roots. Marriage had worked well for them, after all. I'd already been the good wife, the good mother, and, later in my marriage, the black-lingerie whore. To save our marriage, I'd supported my hubby's fantasy of fishnet stockings and frantic sex. And while it saved nothing in the end, the experience did help me realize I prefer the role of dominatrix rather than submissive sex puppet.

Now that I was single and enjoying sex with other men, I found that hand-washing the delicate doilies I was supposed to wear was a chore. And latex had its own set of concerns. So, for my new overnight adventures, I settled on silk camisoles and French-cut underwear. If men wanted a more exotic look, they could wear the sweaty, hot latex themselves.

I was, however, perfectly willing to play with sex toys. For my own pleasure, setting up the scene included candles, wine, music, and sometimes performing the *Dance of the Seven Veils*, each shear layer slowly shed to reveal another silky tease hidden underneath.

My partners always requested the oral item on the *à la carte* menu. But I chose whether to oblige. Since our bodies weren't as limber as they used to be, I often suggested aids to extend the pleasure rather than break a bone. And still, when we were done, there always seemed to be dishes the men wanted doing. Or a wedding they wanted to plan.

I thought I spotted a rare white buffalo at a poetry reading. There he stood in unpretentious jeans, a well-worn leather jacket, and two-day stubble. He even had a faint, appealing look of self-deprecation in his baby-blue eyes. When it was his turn at the mic, he recited a mildly erotic poem, then sat down to drink a cup of herbal tea.

A mix of scruffy punk/hippy with an undertone of gothic romantic, this man was outside the ordinary, so I took a chance and complimented him on his piece, so to speak. When he gave me an enigmatic Mona Lisa smile, I decided he seemed secure enough to accept my bold, and by-now-practiced, invitation. Soon, he became the new lay in my life.

There was no talk of marriage nor need for more than my silky camisole. And where marriage sex had become a stale piece of dry toast, a couple of flips, some crummy bits and a thin spread of arousal, with Mona it was a freshly baked cinnamon roll with layers of sweet spice, soft kisses and sheer indulgence, with no stack of sticky sex manuals needed to show him how.

Could this be true love? Could the rare white buffalo be real? If so, it was not the kind found in fairytales but something honest, without set expectations.

After several weeks of loving Mona, I was delighted when he invited me to his place for dinner, where he both cooked and washed the dishes. Afterwards, we sat to enjoy a game of Boggle (before an anticipated, rousing game of bonking). But as he shook the dice tray, I detected a change. I could feel it coming like the distant rumble of a buffalo herd.

HIM: I'd like to discuss moving forward in our relationship.

ME: Gosh, can we call it a night? I just remembered I have a dental cleaning early tomorrow morning.

HIM: But I need more.

ME: And I need to go.

There had been too many serious discussions in my marriage, and they never changed a thing. Nor did they enhance the mood.

I left poor Mona in the middle of pouring a glass of red wine. *Sorry, beautiful buffalo, but I've been here before*. I guess you're not a miracle after all.

That night, Vic, my trusty vibrator, became the default lay in my life. Vic didn't need candles or music. He supplied nothing but satisfaction. And I didn't even skip all the romance.

Because, just for myself, I performed an abbreviated version of the *Dance of the Seven Veils* in front of my bedroom mirror.

Black Tusk

NICOLA THOMPSON

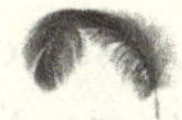

The sun shone brightly against a cerulean sky as I skied off the Peak chairlift at Whistler and laid my eyes upon the impressive Black Tusk in the distance.

I must have been ovulating, because my eyes weren't the only thing I wanted to lay on the Black Tusk. This stunning peak, formed by the leftovers of a long-ago volcano, is an awe-inspiring, dark phallus on the horizon. Seeing it silhouetted against the sky, the first thing that came to mind wasn't the spectacular view, wasn't the beauty of nature; it was a very specific ex-boyfriend's strikingly huge cock.

My quilted green snowpants didn't account for the warmth and swelling in my genitals. The moisture made me feel as though I'd just peed a little bit, and I found myself salivating, as in anticipation of a favorite meal.

The somewhat pleasing, intrusive thought persisted throughout the day, monumental in my mind, just like the Black Tusk. I tried to distract myself with the perfect playlist, then a good book, but nothing worked. All too soon, my attention would return to my nethers. I shuffled in my seat, driving home from the mountain, my thoughts returning to steamy nights on the Prairies, where I'd first connected with Tate. As I reviewed the details in my mind, a flush rose to my cheeks, then wound its way *down there*. (The warmth definitely arose from the inside; my aging and basic little Honda Fit didn't even have a sound system, much less the luxury of heated seats.)

Normally, these feelings wouldn't be an issue. Any aroused thoughts would be purely hypothetical, but . . . Tate had recently moved to the Lower Mainland. This was a problem. Because back when we'd broken up, it had been for very good reasons.

Now he was within driving distance and such passing thoughts—or unpassing as the case was now—were more concerning than back when there were borders between us. It's like having leftover chocolate cake on the counter. It's not nearly the same as just thinking about it when it's still in the store.

The playlist didn't work, the book didn't work, and so I reached out to my friend Ben for a healthy distraction. He'd been my go-to good-times guy and shoulder to cry on since the summer on the sound when we'd signed up for kite-boarding lessons together. We'd play all day in the ocean and debrief how good it was afterwards in the hot tub. We'd soak in the hot water— spent, joyous, and satiated. "It's like sex," we'd agree.

Ben and I also kept each other company through what felt like the weekly break-ups of our late thirties. There wasn't much I'd change about that friendship, except that he was so attractive and straight-passing that he'd regularly, unwittingly, cock-block me. When on the hunt, I'd try to make it very clear that he and I were not an item.

I'm sure Ben sensed the urgency in my voice, because he arrived five minutes after my emergency phone-a-friend, last-ditch-distraction phone call. He picked me up in his much nicer, much faster car and we went downtown for dinner. Unfortunately, Squamish's tiny downtown was too small to provide much distraction either, and our cruise of the main drag was, as usual, disappointing.

Ben and I spent an hour catching up on the usual things: work, skiing, life, but as he drove me back toward my place, we strayed into dangerous territory.

"So . . . you seeing anyone these days?" I asked.

"I wish! Dry spell over here. God, what I wouldn't give for an epic lay."

I laughed. "Is everything okay? You *never* have dry spells!"

That's all it took to break the seal and lead us down the dark path of past loves, lovers, and our strangest, most memorable and—unfortunately—most mind-blowing sex-capades, like the time I moved to Berkeley and took on a lover by referral (seems that's how they do it in Northern California). Unfortunate but unsurprising that we went there, because on ovulation day, all roads lead back to that one thing.

Chats like this weren't unusual for us, a very eligible gay man and his single gal pal, swapping stories and suddenly feeling thirsty. But on this day, I had wound myself up so tight, I was nearly dying of dehydration. While Ben went into steaming, graphic detail about a few of the more exceptional lovers of his recent past, I shuffled around on his slick leather bucket seat.

My mind kept tracing over various parts of Tate's anatomy, and the impact on my body was getting harder and harder to hide. I'm sure if police had pulled over Ben's fast car in that moment, they'd have found a very aroused redhead in the passenger seat, almost panting, pupils fully dilated.

Impossible to contain myself a moment longer, I

blurted this all out to Ben. "I can't stand it! I can't stop thinking about his cock! I blame you, Ben!"

"Dude. Just call the guy. He'll be stoked."

"I mean, what could possibly go wrong?"

Ben raised his eyebrows and gave me one of his most suggestive lopsided smiles.

I giggled, but I also knew how dangerous it was to plant this particular seed. Everything could go wrong.

For one, I could catch feelings, and it had already taken me ages to get over getting under this guy. For another, as an entrepreneur, I no longer had extended health benefits, so what was I supposed to do if I needed another pelvic floor physio appointment?

But I still wanted his body.

The problem was, as much as I wanted Tate's cock right then, I didn't really want the rest of him. During our relationship, there were a lot of things I grew to quite dislike outside of the fire in the bedroom. Most notably, I had struggled with the depth of the debt he'd dug himself into by buying T-shirts and drugs; his desire to move into my place rent-free had really tipped the scales in the end.

Still, his physical attributes were magnetic. That was never the problem. Far from it, actually (though his penis did present some *huge* problems). It was his cock that had previously placed me on the crunchy-white-paper-sheeted examining table of a pelvic floor physiotherapist with her hands up my hoo-haa at 8:00 am on a Tuesday in the first month of our relationship.

The sex had been mind-blowing. Orgasmic in ways I never thought possible. The kind of sex that transports you to another plane of existence. Back then, when I went deep into details with my closest pal, Michelle, though, she said, "Yeah, but it's really more about your connection to the person than their physical traits or some talent they have in bed, right?"

I listened to her politely, but I knew she was wrong. The truth was, Tate had an exceptionally large penis, and he really knew how to use it. I'm talking dangerously long dong, more horse than human. At that time, I'd easily have named him the best lover of my life (as I found myself doing that fateful evening with Ben).

Nothing I tried got Tate's cock off my mind. I kept coming back to it, the way I would to the cookie jar after midnight, padding downstairs barefoot, skipping the squeaky step and hoping no one would catch me.

Ben and I were almost back at my place when, in a desperate final attempt at salvation, I thought of the ice cream shop.

"Hey Ben! Mind dropping me off at the DQ instead? I need a Blizzard."

"Ha! I know what you're up to."

He dropped me off.

"Say hi to Tate for me!" he called out the window as he squealed out of the parking lot.

Shaking my head, I went in and ordered a large Skor Blizzard with Reese's Pieces and extra chocolate fudge sauce.

I ran my tongue around and around my red plastic ice cream spoon, seeking satisfaction, when I suddenly remembered the vibrator I'd recently ordered. My brain is like that: it's not unusual that chocolate peanut-butter ice cream can make me think of vibrators. The connection is pleasure, obviously. ADHD is just like that sometimes. But not to worry if you can't keep up. Most can't, unless they're neurodivergent, too.

The vibrator I'd ordered was one of those rabbit-types, with two ears and a nose, positioned just perfectly (or so I hoped) as to provide maximum satisfaction. I made a deal with myself: if it's there when I get home, I won't text Tate.

Even with all the extras, the Blizzard didn't work. It left me with a stomach ache, still unsatisfied. I walked home from Dairy Queen, shuffling slightly, now contending not only with the swelling between my thighs, but my unhappy belly.

Did I mention I was ovulating? To distract myself, I

put on a guided meditation as I walked: no dice. Tried to call another friend, and again, just found my mind going straight back to my throbbing labia.

I clenched my thighs a little closer, but that just made it worse. I began to wonder whether my arousal was obvious to passers-by. Could they see the way I was waddling? Did the flush in my cheeks give away my desperate craving for sex?

There! *Sex*. Just thinking it again, I'm immediately turned on.

After the bargain I'd made with myself about the vibrator, I felt totally dejected when, upon my arrival home, I saw a long, rectangular cardboard box waiting on my doorstep like a taunt. Once inside my apartment, I opened the package and sat on my bed. I looked at the plastic rabbit for one second, then texted Tate.

How far away are you? I have a bit of a problem.

Instant ping on my phone.

An hour and a half. Are you okay?

I'm totally fine, I was just hoping you were around. I can't stop thinking about . . . [eggplant emoji]

I'll be there in an hour.

When the doorbell rang at midnight, I met Tate with a hug, like I hadn't, an hour earlier, implied I wanted his cock. Never having done this before, I had no idea how to behave. What are the protocols for booty calls?

"Do you want tea?" I asked.

"Seriously?" Tate raised his brows and laughed, gently mocking.

"Tea isn't quite what I had in mind."

And then we got to the point.

For the rest of the night, Tate and I did everything we used to do. Even this one thing I'm not going to tell you about.

But do you know what? It did nothing for me.

Sex with Tate that night wasn't remotely as I'd remembered. At one point, I even wondered, *Is it in?*

I actually couldn't tell. I felt numb to the very same cock I'd dreamed about and glorified for the past five years. I felt no connection to Tate and could barely feel myself there in the bed beside him. (Note: the size of his penis had not changed since the last time I slept with him. Obviously.)

Afterwards, tangled in sheets and sweating but still not satisfied, I realized that Michelle had—as she usually, annoyingly was—been right. I'd assumed her to be sexually naive at the time, but she already knew something I didn't. (I've since conducted my fair share of field research. When it comes to sex, if the connection isn't there for me, nothing is.)

That trash message (origin: patriarchy) that I used to believe, that says it's better for men to have bigger cocks is not just judgmental, but also totally, and harmfully, wrong.

And so, well, sometimes, it turns out that doing the crazy thing and just buying a second ice cream really is the healthier choice.

Just ask my pelvic floor physio.

Contributors

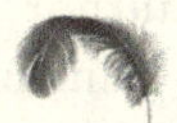

The daughter of a narcissistic former pastor who didn't leave her fear-driven worldviews until her 40s, **Andrea Andres** is learning to validate her own way of existing past performance-based love. She teaches her children to embrace their own sexual ethic while simultaneously understanding how to manage her asexuality after more than twenty years of marriage. She lives in Squamish, BC.

Jade Francesca Bartlett is a queer, neurodivergent artist who marries the vulnerable with the ferocious in everything she creates. Jade is not only a writer, but a multidisciplinary actress and photographer. When she is not creating, she is dreaming of all the things she wishes to create in the future!

Nicole Breit is a multi-award-winning essayist based in Gibsons, BC and the co-author of *Bloom: Letters on Girlhood* (Caitlin Press, 2025). She is a narrative therapy trained writing coach and the founder of Spark Your

Story, a series of programs for emerging and seasoned creative nonfiction writers. Visit her at nicolebreit.com.

Sarah Byrd is a therapist, photographer, and founder of *still / space Branding & Photography* that serves clinical counselors. Her expertise spans Buddhism, transpersonal psychology, therapeutic photography, and past life regressions. She's the author of *Unfolding: Therapy Companion Journal* and splits her time between Denver, Colorado, and Austin, Texas.

Hannah Davis is a Canadian-born nonfiction writer and confidence coach. After years of masking and running from her truth, she finally broke—setting fire to her old life. Now proudly queer, Hannah's raw unfiltered stories crack open taboo topics around money, sex, shame, and identity. Her forthcoming memoir, *Sugar Hit,* is a bold reclamation of power, pleasure, and self-worth.

Based in Squamish, BC, and hailing from rural Quebec, **Pierre-Olivier Gaudreault** is a writer, mountain athlete and active traveling guide. His first non-fiction story appeared in *Awfully Hilarious: Stories We Never Tell* (2023). Passionate about people and connection, he blends vulnerability and humor to capture unspoken experiences, helping people connect through shared stories of life and adventure.

Geoffrey K. Graves has been widely published and honored internationally. Pushcart Nominee (US–2023/4);

Finalist, Cutthroat Barry Lopez Nonfiction Award (US–2019); Winner, Grindstone Literary Anthology (UK–2020); Finalist, Tobias Wolff Award (US–2021); Shortlist, Bath Flash Fiction Award (Ireland–2021); 2nd place, Periscope Literary (UK–2022); Three Honorable Mentions Writers Digest (US–2023); One of three winners, McClaren Memorial Comedy Festival One-Act Play Competition (US–2025). Employed Script Department at CBS Television City, Hollywood. MFA California State University, Fullerton. He lives in Palm Springs, California.

Heather Hendrie is a nature-based therapist, clinical counsellor and writer who founded the Awfully Hilarious Project to end shame, uplift women's health and destigmatize mental health. She is based in Whistler, BC.

kate heskett (they/them) is an award-winning poet, writer and canoe guide. Their short stories have been published in *Pique* newsmagazine and the *Lupine Review*. They are forever working on their first novel.

Yin Xzi Ho (何吟曦) is an author and artist with a focus on land-based practices and knowledge. Born in Kuala Lumpur, Malaysia, and now based in Squamish, Canada, her work is inspired by the places she has been. Yin Xzi's other publications include a memoir, *Home Is Here*. She is also a live typewriter poet at events for friends and strangers where she tries to render the magic that often goes unseen from our smallest and most significant moments of everyday life in order to touch the hearts of the people around her.

Angelina Jimenez is an author, ancestral healer, and community advocate based in California's Bay Area. She was first published at seven years old in an anthology for young authors and has been writing ever since.

Dean Slugger Jones (he/they) is a writer, yoga teacher, and body worker in Hudson, New York. His writing is an emotional deep dive into longing, trans identity, queer desire, intimacy, sex, and grief. You can find his words in *New Words Press* (Issue 6), *Not Ghosts, But Spirits V* (Querencia Press), *Identity Theory* magazine, and *The Anatomy of Breakup Sex* (Wet Press).

Simarbir Kaur is an IT professional by the day and an ardent book lover by the night. Through her Bookstagram she spotlights books and authors, and loves to recommend books, write insightful reviews and post creative bookish content. Simar lives in Whitby, Ontario with her husband and two children. She can be reached at @simar.bookish.dreamer (IG)

Claire Locey moves between feminist thought and everyday wonder. With a BA in Gender and Women's Studies and a Master's in Community Health Sciences, she sees stories as ways of knowing and acts of resistance. Joy finds her paddling a canoe with her husband or walking her black lab, Ducky. She lives in Calgary, Alberta.

Sophia McGovern is a writer living in Tempe, Arizona, with her husband, new baby, and cat. She is the founding editor of Little Somethings Press, which publishes flash fiction, flash memoir, poetry, and art in handmade books. Her work has appeared in *Motherlore Magazine*, Fiction Attic Press, and other places.

Achiro P. Olwoch is a Ugandan writer, playwright, and storyteller whose work explores exile, memory, queerness, and postcolonial identity. She holds an MFA in Creative Writing from Lasell University and has written plays and prose that center strong African voices. She lives in Poughkeepsie, New York, where she writes across stage and page.

Wendy L. Schmidt lives in Appleton, Wisconsin. She is the published author of short stories, poetry and essays. She is also a mixed media artist as well as the creator of short poetry films.

Claire Sicherman is the author of *Bloom: Letters on Girlhood* (a collaboration with Nicole Breit) and *Imprint: A Memoir of Trauma in the Third Generation*. Her writing has been featured in acclaimed anthologies and literary journals. As a facilitator, speaker, and trauma-informed somatic coach, Claire supports brave humans in bringing the stories they hold in their bodies onto the page. Find her at: clairesicherman.com.

Anastasia Soroka is an author, certified trauma therapist, and host of the podcast *Insights with Us*. Her dream is to build a community of like-minded people who embody acceptance and authenticity. In her free time, you can find her cuddling with her dog, climbing, or getting lost in nature.

Nicola Thompson (she/they) isn't shy about the body's hungriest desires. Her latest work teases apart the erotic charge of ovulation, all heat and honesty. She's currently circling Whistler, where the mountains aren't the only things rising.

Gratitude

A project like this is such a privilege. Writing and working alongside our courageous crew of contributors tops the list as one of the best parts of it all. For all of you who stepped up to share your stories (whether they made it onto these pages or not), we thank you!

To our editor Darcie Friesen-Hossack, thanks for all you've done to make these stories sing.

Shout out to our all the donors and supporters who made this community-supported project possible, and of course to our 69th backer, who climaxed our Kickstarter campaign.

Endless gratitude to Stella Harvey and her ongoing legacy with the Whistler Writers' Society for supporting a healthy and growing ecosystem of writers.

And of course to you, the reader: where these pages touch your palms is where the magic happens. We can't do it without you.

Thanks to The Canada Council for The Arts, for funding our accompanying audiobook. If you want to hear these stories in each writer's own words (highly recommend), stream our *Pillow Talk* audiobook anywhere you listen to books.

Thanks again for being here.

xo Angelina & Heather

About the awfully hilarious project

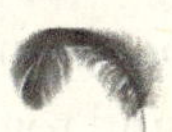

We are so glad you're here.

At its outset, the awfully hilarious idea grew out of a bad date, the subsequent call to a dear friend who'd also just returned from a dismal date, and the exasperated/joking statement, "We could write a book!"

And it very quickly then took on a life of its own. While the initial stories we gathered together focused on disastrous dating experiences and mortifying bodily function moments, they very quickly expanded to encompass women's health, medical mishaps, struggles with fertility, and beyond.

After our first book, *Stories We Never Tell*, came out, suddenly, people began to get in touch with us to share their stories. As the stories of embarrassment, shame, and fear flowed in, we recognized that our fun little project had grown bigger than a lark. Folks wanted more than a single-and-dating support group (though we need that too). The awfully hilarious project revealed a growing community yearning to belong, who craved connection—and real talk—on topics that really matter.

We're not the first to do this, and we certainly hope we won't be the last. Our approach is humor. We use laughter to make the poignant and the painful more palatable. We use tears and togetherness to heal.

In shaping each awfully hilarious anthology, we think often about the people who came before us—the ones who whispered their truths in kitchens, bedrooms, locker rooms, and back alleys, long before it was safe to speak openly. The legacy of liberation lives in those quiet acts of bravery. It lives in every moment someone chooses honesty over silence.

What we create here isn't a single narrative, nor a one-size-fits-all version of the human experience. Instead, it's a gathering—a place where people can show up exactly as they are and know that their story matters. Where contradictions are welcome. Where vulnerability is honored. Where humor and heartbreak sit together at the table.

With every anthology, we keep widening the circle. We keep reimagining. We keep centering the voices that have always deserved to be heard, with the space to speak their own words, on their own terms.

In particular, we pay homage to the brilliance of the many Black, Indigenous, trans, queer people of color who paved the way for the tradition of truth-telling. Without artists, activists, and feminists like bell hooks, Audre Lorde, Angela Davis, Kimberlé Crenshaw, Maya Angelou, adrienne maree brown, and so many others, our stigma-smashing stories would most certainly have remained tucked away in our private journals and thoughts or said in secret to our friends or therapists.

Thank you for being here. Thank you for helping us make the awful just a little bit more hilarious. We are so glad to have you join us as we strive to start meaningful, healing conversations, and to shift the narrative together through truth and through story.

Join us on socials @awfullyhilarious.

We can't wait to hear your stories!

www.awfullyhilarious.com

Subscribe to the awfully hilarious newsletter

Submit your story to the awfully hilarious project

awfully hilarious

STORIES WE NEVER TELL

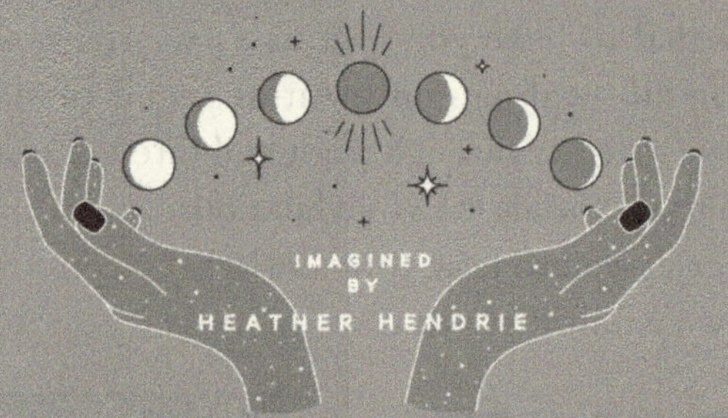

Awfully Hilarious Stories We Never Tell

Omg this book was hysterical! I read this in one sitting and laughed out loud so hard I had to pause as I couldn't see the words for my tears!! An absolute must read!!

~ GOODREADS

If you laughed, gasped, or nodded along, you'll love *Awfully Hilarious Stories We Never Tell*, the book that started it all. From dating disasters, to medical mishaps, to the bodily functions and misadventures that people usually keep to themselves, every story is bold, honest, and utterly relatable.

Readers have called it "hilarious, heartfelt, and impossible to put down"—and now it's your turn to dive in. Come along for the laugh-out-loud moments, submit your own story, join the community, and discover even more hilarity waiting in every page.

And here's the best part: you don't have to keep it to yourself. *Awfully Hilarious: Stories We Never Tell* is the balm for the soul that you're going to want to share with anyone who is disillusioned with dating and needs some company and a good laugh.

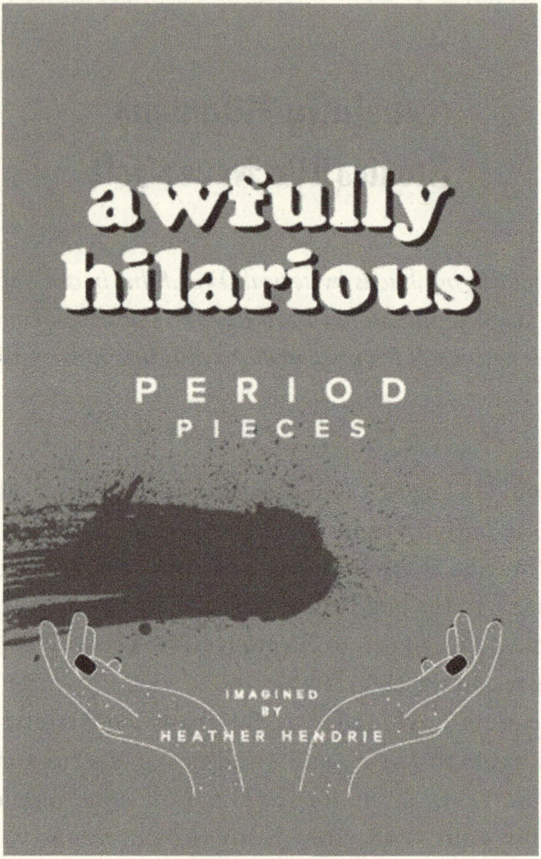

awfully hilarious

PERIOD PIECES

IMAGINED BY HEATHER HENDRIE

Awfully Hilarious Period Pieces

Ready for a bloody good time?

This book laid bare the embarrassing parts of life, the moments that we push under the rug and try to forget about... It turned that shame on its head and made it beautiful.

~GOODREADS

If you're in the midst of a hot flash right now, bring this one with you into the walk-in freezer. *Period Pieces* is a deep dive into the awkward, absurd, and sometimes very messy moments of menstruation—from first menses through to "the pause." These stories offer a range of experiences, from painful and poignant to outright hilarious, that prove you're never alone, and that it's a whole lot easier when we can laugh about it together.

Readers have called this one, "relatable, honest, transformative and the book [they] wish [they'd] had years ago".

Our community is full of readers who share, connect, and write their own stories. Ready to join us? Submit your tale, join the laughter, and explore other books in the series that will keep the hilarity flowing.

You know you want to . . . Leave a review and tell us how much you enjoyed *Pillow Talk!*

Join us at the awfully hilarious project.